ASTHMA:

An Alternative Approach

Ron Roberts and Judy Sammut

Ron Roberts has suffered from asthma since childhood, but has managed to control his condition using the techniques he describes in this book. He has worked with asthmatics in a number of complementary medical fields for many years. He trained first as a teacher, then as a natural therapist, gaining qualifications in naturopathy, chiropractic and acupuncture. He has also run successful swimming programs for asthmatics.

Judy Sammut, who helped to write this book, has a background in public relations.

ASTHMA:
An Alternative Approach

Ron Roberts and Judy Sammut

Keats Publishing, Inc. 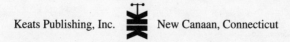 New Canaan, Connecticut

*To my late wife Gwen, who inspired me
with her faith, hope and love.*

RR

Asthma: An Alternative Approach

This edition is published in 1997 by arrangement with Penguin Books Australia Ltd.

Library of Congress Cataloging-in-Publication Data

CIP Information:
Roberts, R.A. (Ronald Alfred), 1934-
    Asthma: an alternative approach/Ron Roberts and Judy Sammut.
        p.   cm.
    Includes bibliographical references and index.
    ISBN 0-87983-771-3
    1. Asthma—Alternative treatment.   I. Sammut, Judy.   II. Title.
RC591.R53   1997
816.2'3806—DC21   96-52334
                                                                        CIP

Printed in United States of America

Published by Keats Publishing, Inc.
27 Pine Street, Box 876
New Canaan, Connecticut 06840-0876

99 98 97 6 5 4 3 2 1

CONTENTS

ACKNOWLEDGMENTS

My sincerest thanks to Judy Sammut. This book would not have been completed without her constructive co-ordination and rewriting of my manuscript.

I would also like to thank my family for their confidence in me and their assistance with the book, my patients, and my teaching associates and fellow practitioners, who have encouraged and supported my philosophy of health and well-being.

Judy and I are indebted to Clare Coney of Viking for her editing expertise in refining these pages.

Ron Roberts

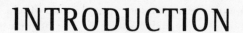

INTRODUCTION

Asthma has slowly but surely been increasing in its incidence over the last few decades, until it can be said without exaggeration to have reached epidemic status in many countries, with one in four children now diagnosed to have it to some degree in certain industrialized societies. Why is this quiet epidemic occurring? No one knows for sure, but it is widely believed that people in the developed world are being exposed to much higher amounts of allergens in their lives than they used to be, and this is related to the rising incidence of asthma.

Asthma is not an inconvenience. It is a potentially lethal condition that has no cure, only medication to lessen the severity and number of attacks. There are thousands of deaths annually as a direct or indirect result of asthma. Many are preventable. Asthma is responsible for more admissions of children to hospitals than any other condition and is the greatest reason for schooldays lost.

These deaths are not generally happening because the asthma is untreated. Statistics show that in some countries asthma medications are now the second largest category of prescriptions dispensed, so conventional medicine is trying its best. Can anything more be done? We believe the answer is "Yes." There are many alternative therapies that do alleviate asthma and there are specific exercises that considerably improve asthmatics' condition. There is also much benefit that can be gained by the asthmatic following a generally healthier way of life.

This book is an attempt to give the reader as much

----

information as possible: about asthma itself, the exercises Ron has found most helpful over decades of working with people with asthma, and natural therapies and treatments for it that are presently available. It is our hope that asthmatics will thus better understand what may be causing their condition, and may pursue avenues of treatment that will improve their health.

Unfortunately the holistic view of health is regarded with suspicion by many people, as it does not rely on technological intervention in the body which can be measured and controlled. It is difficult to demonstrate repeatable results using many alternative therapies. This does not mean they do not work – but they may work better for some people than others. You can only try the therapies yourself and see if your asthma improves.

Orthodox medicine and complementary medicine have different approaches to treating asthma. But there should be no controversy about who is right or who is wrong. For the sake of asthmatics we feel it would be far better if a spirit of cooperation and collaboration existed instead. Asthma management should encompass all aspects of a person and his condition.

As the book discusses many different methods of healing, readers will probably not have heard of some of these therapies before. This does not mean that they are new or revolutionary. Most natural therapies have been used for decades, often centuries, and although some may have become neglected there has been a resurgence of interest recently in traditional approaches. We make no apologies for including esoteric or unusual therapies in this book; they may not, at present, have scientific acceptance, but twenty years ago neither did acupuncture and chiropractic, which are widely used today by medical practitioners.

A Personal View

Ron has been a severe asthmatic since childhood so asthma has always been a part of his life. Ron remembers: "My father suffered from asthma, constantly wheezing and being extremely short of breath. I can vividly recall when I was about fourteen how my father would hold his head over a metal pie dish with burning asthma powder in it. A very popular asthma remedy then, this powder contained a variety of herbs (including marijuana and belladonna) plus creosote, and could be readily purchased in pharmacies. My father would light the powder, bend over and inhale the fumes given off. He did this every morning.

"When I was twenty-one he was prescribed different medication, but remained faithful to the powder. He eventually found relief by natural means when he was introduced late in life to a particular breathing technique.

"I remember my first asthma attack vividly. I was eight. Suddenly I could not get my breath. I was rushed to the hospital, where a mask was put over my face. Subsequently I had to take tablets two or three times a day, and carry these with me constantly. I also used an atomizer that discharged asthma powder into my mouth when I squeezed the rubber bulb. Despite the medication, asthma attacks and wheezing were a daily part of my life into adulthood. I am sure most asthmatics will have similar stories.

"When I was about thirty I decided to be more positive about my asthma, and to try various therapies to see if I could improve my health. The breathing technique that had helped my father also helped me, and a relapse when I did not have the determination to persevere convinced me of its benefits.

"However, after returning to my alternative treatment program – and expanding it – my asthma abated. I came to the conclusion that a radical change of attitude in my life was necessary: I needed to be aware that everything I did would have an effect upon my asthma. I became interested in alternative medicine, and trained in various disciplines – naturopathy, chiropractic, acupuncture, Chinese medicine, homeopathy, herbal medicine, massage and German high-tech bio-energetic medicine. My health has improved so much that I completed a full marathon when I was forty-five, when previously I could not run 500 meters without wheezing, coughing or setting off a severe attack. I have had no need to take any prescribed drugs for many years."

This holistic view of health and asthma is central to this book: asthma has many causes, and many treatments may bring relief. Overall, though, the asthmatic's goal should be to build up resistance to asthma, and strengthen his or her body's immune system.

Combining Orthodox and Alternative Medicine

Although this book is primarily concerned with natural remedies, and improving asthma through alternative treatments, we do not underestimate the value of orthodox medication. Medication such as Ventolin, Vanceril or cortisone may be of help, especially when the asthma is acute, because these drugs bring immediate relief. **In an emergency your prescribed medication should always be used**, as alternative approaches work towards long-term prevention of asthma rather than immediate relief in an attack.

Neither orthodox medicine nor alternative therapies can cure asthma. Both can only control it. However, it is our belief that if people with asthma persevere with the suggestions in this book, their condition will quickly and significantly improve, and may even reach a stage where they can describe it as under control without needing to use drugs.

Do not expect immediate results from following alternative therapies: improvement will take a little time, and may require major changes to your lifestyle. You should use these alternative methods as well as your prescribed medication, **not** instead of, and explain to your doctor what you are doing. The aim of this book is to help you manage your asthma more effectively, and be able to lessen your reliance on drugs once the asthma has improved.

Because asthma is caused by many factors there is no single remedy for it. The most effective treatments will be different for everybody. Do not dismiss an idea in the following chapters because you do not think it will work for you. Keep an open mind.

NOTE We have chosen to include in this book descriptions of some treatments that appear to have limited effects when treating asthma. They are here because alternative practitioners may recommend them to their asthmatic patients, and thus asthmatics may wish to find out more about them. Inclusion in this book does not mean that we necessarily recommend them.

PART ONE

BEING AN
ASTHMATIC

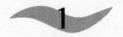

WHAT IS ASTHMA?

Asthma, essentially, is a condition where the sufferer has difficulty breathing. The word **asthma** is derived from the Greek word meaning panting or breathing hard. Wheezing and shortness of breath are the most obvious symptoms during an attack.

The commonly seen type of asthma is bronchial asthma. It is caused by a narrowing of the passages that carry air from the throat to the lungs. This narrowing can be due to muscle contraction, local inflammation or the production of excess mucus. The result is the same: difficulty in breathing. Wheezing is often heard as the asthmatic person breathes out. The recommendations in this book are aimed at sufferers of bronchial asthma of all kinds.

Another, uncommon, type of asthma is called cardiac asthma. It is a symptom of heart disease, where the heart is not pumping the blood around the body strongly enough to deliver sufficient oxygen to the muscles. The body's response is to try to increase the uptake of oxygen by bringing more air into the lungs; a feeling of breathlessness results. Cardiac asthma should only be treated by medical practitioners.

The Respiratory System

The respiratory system is the name given to the lungs and all the passages that bring air from the environment down into the body.

Diaphragm function.

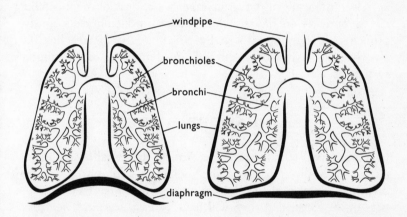

Breathing out: diaphragm contracts   Breathing in: diaphragm descends

In normal breathing, outward movement of the rib cage and downward movement of the diaphragm together draw air into the lungs via the windpipe (trachea); the trachea divides into two bronchi that themselves divide into smaller branches, the bronchioles. These lead to grape-like sacs in the lungs, the alveoli.

The walls of the alveolar sacs are thin and well supplied with tiny blood vessels. Oxygen taken into the alveolar sacs moves into the red blood cells in the walls and carbon dioxide is released by these red blood cells into the lungs. The diaphragm and rib cage then contract simultaneously, forcing air out of the lungs, and the person breathes out. In a healthy individual all this happens without conscious control.

The amount of air taken into the lungs is also varied automatically when you breathe. The bronchi are made of

----

muscles and these can expand or contract. The nervous system can change the width of the bronchi, and when all is working well the bronchi will expand when more air is needed (during intense exercise, for instance) and contract when there is little demand for oxygen by the body (such as when you are asleep).

The air coming into the lungs is also regulated: its temperature and humidity are adjusted to ensure that the maximum amount of oxygen can be extracted from it by the alveoli. Blood vessels in the walls of the air passages warm or cool the incoming air to body temperature, while mucus-producing cells in the bronchi add humidity to it. By the time the air reaches the alveolar sacs it has been through the body's 'air conditioning' system!

An Asthma Attack

In a bronchial asthma attack the bronchi do not allow sufficient air to reach the lungs, and the individual begins to labor for breath. In a typical attack the sufferer will first feel a tightness in the chest and then will have to gasp for air. They may start wheezing or coughing. The face may turn gray-blue – particularly around the nose and mouth. The sufferer may feel a need for fresh air and may try to open all doors and windows. In a severe attack the brain will not be receiving enough oxygen to function properly and the asthmatic may become muddled or disoriented.

Most attacks are mild and will last no more than an hour. Sometimes the asthma improves after the patient coughs up a considerable amount of mucus. However, untreated attacks may last for days and the effects can be severe and dangerous.

If you suspect that you, or a member of your family, may have asthma you should discuss this with your doctor. When the diagnosis is asthma you will usually be given a prescription for a pharmaceutical drug to be taken during attacks and may also be prescribed a preventative that is taken regularly to keep airway inflammation to a minimum. You should use medication whenever an asthma attack occurs. If the condition is severe and does not respond to home treatment you should contact your doctor; in an emergency, go to the hospital emergency room or call an ambulance.

The recommendations in Part Two of this book are long-term strategies to lessen the likelihood of asthma attacks occurring, but they are not intended to replace orthodox treatment during an attack. **Asthma attacks must always be treated promptly with prescribed medication**.

STATUS ASTHMATICUS

This is a medical term meaning a very severe and prolonged asthma attack. There is extreme difficulty in breathing and exhaustion and collapse may follow. Hospitalization is almost always necessary and close monitoring is required. Status asthmaticus is life-threatening.

Never ignore an asthma attack in the hope that it will go away by itself. Status asthmaticus may well be the result.

CHRONIC ASTHMA

Asthma affects people in different ways. It can appear in childhood or during adulthood; worsen gradually or have a sudden onset. Some people may have only one attack in their entire life, but for others asthma is a chronic condition.

Where the asthma is chronic the bronchial tubes may be narrower than normal, and since generally asthma treatment is aimed at increasing their width to allow more air to pass through, treating chronic asthma may be more difficult than treating acute asthma. Chronic asthmatics may also have chronic overproduction of mucus in their bronchi, making the situation worse.

Other Respiratory Disorders

There are a number of respiratory disorders that have symptoms similar to asthma, and they may be confused with asthma. The similarities can lead to the assumption that a person is suffering from asthma when any shortness of breath occurs.

There is a danger that asthma is being overdiagnosed at present. A thorough medical examination is essential if asthma is suspected, to ensure the exact condition is determined and treatments are not prescribed unnecessarily.

BRONCHITIS
Bronchitis is an inflammation of the bronchi or bronchioles, in which excess mucus is produced. This causes a cough and breathing difficulties. The bronchitis can be the result of an infection such as a cold or flu, or irritation by foreign substances, particularly tobacco smoke and air pollution. ,

The condition can be acute – of fairly short duration – or chronic, when it can lead to emphysema. Chronic bronchitis may be treated medically using some of the same drugs that are prescribed for asthma, as the aim in both cases is to reduce the production of mucus and increase the flow of air through the bronchi.

CROUP
Croup is most often caused by a virus but can also be the result of certain bacterial infections or a severe allergy. During a croup attack the air passage at the entrance to the larynx narrows. Breathing becomes difficult and is accompanied by a harsh cough.

Mostly affecting infants and small children, this acute respiratory infection usually comes on at night and can be frightening for both child and parent. Repeated attacks of croup can occur over two or three successive nights.

EMPHYSEMA
Emphysema is a very serious condition in which the alveolar sacs in the lungs are enlarged and damaged beyond repair. The sacs lose their elasticity, grow larger, and no longer function efficiently at exchanging the oxygen and carbon dioxide gases between the lungs and bloodstream. The body does not receive sufficient oxygen and the immediate symptoms of emphysema are therefore similar to asthma: shortness of breath, wheeziness and often bluish-gray colored skin. Additionally there is a chronic cough that brings up sticky sputum or mucus.

As the condition worsens the patient has increased difficulty breathing and may need to be given oxygen through a mask.

The Diagnosis of Asthma

Asthma should always be thoroughly diagnosed, and it is important that the **cause** is understood. Many people with asthma think they know what is causing it, but they may not necessarily be correct, and unless they have had a proper assessment of their triggers the asthma may not be treated properly, and the condition will not be managed effectively.

A medical practitioner will first take details of your history, and then may carry out diagnostic tests. He or she will certainly listen to your chest using a stethoscope, through which the sounds you make while breathing are amplified. If the asthma seems to be mild the doctor may then give you a prescription to use when necessary. However, if the condition appears to be more severe further tests may be carried out.

- A spirometer is a machine that measures lung capacity, and is capable of giving a reasonably accurate indication of the severity of the asthma. It is often used to check on improvement or decline in breathing function. Alternatively a simple peak flow meter may be used to check lung capacity. Peak flow meters are often used in the home (see pages 25–6).
- X-rays: an experienced radiologist may be able to detect changes in the bronchi and bronchioles that are indicative of asthma, and chest X-rays will also rule out the possibility of another disease causing the symptoms.
- CT, or computerized tomography, scanning is being used more and more to diagnose asthma. Essentially it is a combination of X-ray and computer technology that allows a three-dimensional picture to be built up of tissues of the body, particularly soft tissues such as lungs, which do not show up so well on X-rays.
- Skin tests can show whether the asthmatic is allergic to any specific substances that may be triggering attacks. Skin prick tests are usually painless. A drop of allergic extract is placed on the skin surface and a prick made at the same spot with a needle. If a small, itchy hive appears within ten to twenty minutes it indicates a positive reaction – an allergy – to that substance.

- Pathology tests of sputum and blood are sometimes
  carried out to confirm asthma, and urine samples can
  also be analyzed. A full blood examination (FBE) will
  reveal possible allergic reactions (if a particular type of
  white blood cell is present in greater than normal
  numbers) and further RAST blood tests (radioallergosorbent test or radio-allergenic sensitivity test)
  identify individual allergies. RAST measures the specific
  antibodies in the blood serum to a particular allergen
  and is often used in place of skin testing.

  Sputum discoloration can be caused by asthma or be
  the result of an infection or allergy so a sputum analysis
  may be carried out. This is not standard practice,
  however, and the information that can be deduced from
  such tests is not accepted in all medical circles.

There are further tests that may be suggested by natural
therapists, depending on their speciality. Although these
may confirm the presence of asthma you should not rely on
them as the only diagnosis of your condition.

- Spinal diagnosis involves X-rays, palpation or using a
  two-pronged thermometer to measure the difference in
  temperature between the sides of the spine.

Spinal diagnosis using two-pronged thermometer.

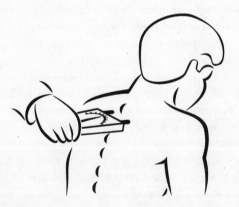

- Iris diagnosis: practitioners use lesions, colorings and blemishes in the iris of the eye to make a diagnosis. Iridology was based on the theories of a Hungarian surgeon, Ignatz von Peczely, but has been developed by several leading iridologists. Particular areas of the iris are considered to be related to parts of the body, and sickness in an organ will show itself as markings in that section of the iris.
- Chinese medicine uses changes in the pulse rate to determine whether the patient has a particular condition.
- Southeast Asian practitioners may use tongue diagnosis to assess the health of the patient.

There are also lesser known methods of diagnosing asthma, which must be considered to be of dubious value.

- Hair sampling: hairs from your head are examined under a microscope to make a diagnosis.
- VEGA testing, in which the electrical conductivity in your body is measured by machine. VEGA testing is also used to detect allergies.
- SEG (segmental electrograph) testing: a diagnostic method in which segments of the body are stimulated in turn. The SEG machine gives readings that indicate how the parts of the body react to this mild stimulus and from them a diagnosis may be made.
- Some people claim that latent asthma can be detected by signs in the palm of the hand. We cannot recommend this as a means of diagnosis!

Once a proper diagnosis has been made of the asthma and its severity, your doctor may suggest further monitoring of the condition at home. Usually a peak flow meter is used, and further details are given in Chapter 3.

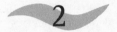

WHAT CAUSES
ASTHMA?

Asthma and other respiratory complaints are known to affect approximately one out of every six people in most industrialized societies. The primary cause of asthma is unknown and there are as many theories about its causes as there are "cures." However, in the past few years we have discovered a good deal about what sets off asthma.

Statistically, parents who have asthma are more likely to have asthmatic children than nonasthmatic parents. However, the link is not simple, as parents who have a history of allergies in general – food allergies, eczema and hives, for instance – are also more likely to have asthmatic children than nonallergy-prone parents. The conclusion drawn from this is that asthma may be linked in some way to the general immune response of the body, and that there is a genetic factor: it is passed from parent to child. Repeated studies have supported this evidence, but that does not mean all asthma is hereditary, as many people develop asthma without any allergic history themselves or in their immediate family.

Research groups have been trying to pin down the "asthma gene" in susceptible families by analyzing their chromosomes (the long strings of genetic material in the nuclei of cells that carry the genes). The idea is that members of the family who have asthma or allergies should be carrying a gene that nonallergic relatives do not have. A group of scientists in Oxford believe they have isolated the gene responsible on Chromosome 11. The most recent research shows that genes may also be linked to "airway twitchiness" (see page 13) as well as allergic responses.

Knowing where an allergy gene is (and there may be more than one, still to be found) does not, however, mean that at present asthma or allergies can be reliably prevented from developing. There is hope, though. If in the future an easy test is developed that shows whether or not someone is carrying the gene, sufferers would be able to minimize exposure to potential allergens that might set off the condition.

Chest infection is often the cause of asthma in people who do not have any allergic symptoms. Their asthma may recur whenever they are ill, but is not linked to environmental factors.

Finally, emotional upsets and stress can cause asthma.

Patterns of Asthma

Few babies are born with asthma but it can develop at any time of life – although it usually does so in childhood rather than in adult years. Asthma is seldom serious in infants but tends to become more severe through childhood, generally worsening around 8–14 years of age. Males are more likely to develop asthma than females, for reasons not understood at present.

The most common cause of infant asthma is a virus infection, but in children up to the teenage years house dust and pets do the damage, followed in adulthood by pollens and molds. Over 45 years of age, chemical-based irritants, infections and cold air take over as primary causes of asthma.

The pattern of childhood asthma often changes in adolescence, as a child may simply "grow out of" the complaint during his or her teenage years. This is not always the case though, and children who have been asthmatics are always at risk of having attacks in adult life if exposed to a sufficiently strong trigger. For a minority of asthmatic children – about one in five – the asthma will in fact worsen through adolescence and into adulthood.

A typical asthmatic will more than likely have had an early medical history of frequent colds, allergic conditions, sinusitis, hay fever, eczema, bronchial complaints, influenza and low resistance to a range of diseases. This is to be expected if asthma is linked to the immune system, as will be explained later.

Having said that, there are plenty of cases where adults have suddenly developed asthma without any prior warning. The onset is often linked to some change in their circumstances, such as moving house or changing jobs, which brings them in contact with an allergen that they had not been exposed to before. Attacks of asthma have been found to be more common during puberty, times of emotional stress, menstruation, pregnancy and menopause, all of which point to emotional or hormonal factors playing a part. Asthma is also more likely to occur if the person is fatigued or is undertaking strenuous physical activity.

What Happens During an Attack

How does being allergic cause asthma? Why do some people get asthma from changes in temperature or humidity – surely people aren't allergic to weather? There are many aspects of asthma that may seem quite puzzling.

As explained in Chapter 1, during an asthma attack the air passages to the lungs become smaller, making it difficult for the asthmatic to get sufficient air. This may be caused by three factors, and often a combination of all three occurs in an attack.

Variation in airways causing asthma.

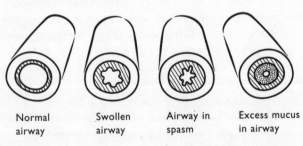

| Normal airway | Swollen airway | Airway in spasm | Excess mucus in airway |

- The walls of the passages may have swollen due to inflammation.
- The passages may have gone into spasm as the muscles in and around their walls contract.
- Some asthmatics produce excess mucus, which clogs the air passages further.

The result is the same: reduced size of the air passages, and reduced flow of air to the lungs, with the symptoms of asthma.

INFLAMMATION

Inflammation may be difficult to visualize in the airways, but compare it to what happens when you have a sprained ankle or wrist: that part of your body swells up. The swelling can happen rapidly, and doesn't necessarily mean there is an infection. What it does mean is that the body has mobilized its defense system, the white blood cells, to go to the site where there is a problem.

In an asthma attack caused by an allergen the air passages to the lungs send a message to the defense system that they have encountered some potentially dangerous substance in the air. White blood cells respond by moving to the airways. The passage walls swell as a result, making it difficult to breathe. A non-asthmatic will not have the same problem, as his or her body will not recognize the trigger particle (be it pollen, dust mite material or other allergen) as dangerous. People with asthma are allergic to it, and their bodies overreact.

BRONCHIAL SPASM

Bronchial spasm is also called "airway twitchiness." It is what happens when the muscles surrounding the air passages receive a nerve signal to contract. This may be part of the allergic response – the body trying to protect the lungs from the allergen it has encountered by closing down the air passages – or it may be non-allergenic, and a simple response by the respiratory system to the inhalation of an irritant particle. It may be the reaction of the body to sudden cold air, or changes in humidity. It may also be the result of an infection, where the body is more sensitive than usual to the particles being inhaled. Whatever the cause, it is the muscle and nerve systems in the lungs over-reacting, instead of the white blood cells' defense system.

EXCESS MUCUS

Excess mucus secretion can happen in a number of infections, particularly bronchitis and cold viruses, or as the body's response to an inhaled irritant or allergen.

Forms of Asthma

Because asthma is the end result of the body reacting in different ways to different stimuli, doctors categorize the various asthma types.

1 Allergic (or atopic or extrinsic) asthma, which is asthma caused by allergens, often dust mites or pollen.
2 Nonallergic asthma, often triggered by infection or pollution.
3 Asthma resulting from emotional or physical situations.
4 Intrinsic asthma, a chronic asthma not triggered by allergies and with no obvious cause but often seen in adult-onset rather than in childhood asthma.

In fact, many asthma attacks will be the result of a combination of two or even all four types. An inhaled substance may be an allergen and cause inflammation, but it may also be perceived as an irritant and result in bronchial spasm. Finally, when asthmatics realize they are having an attack they may panic, thus setting off more spasms through emotional and hormonal triggers. It is difficult to distinguish between the types of asthma attack in practice, so it is wise for people with asthma to know what causes their particular attacks, so they may minimize them.

Allergic Asthma

Allergies are the result of the body reacting to a substance as if it was a dangerous disease particle and trying to attack it with the white blood cells.

If a virus or bacterium gets into our bloodstream the white blood cells have an important role in fighting the invader. They "recognize" that the outer surface of the virus or bacterium is foreign and make a mirror copy of it. The mirror image, or template, is then used as a blueprint to make hundreds of thousands of white blood cells that are specifically designed to attack that surface. These cells are carried through the bloodstream and whenever they encounter the particular surface they are programmed against – the infection – they destroy it.

This defense system is a great way of keeping viruses and bacteria at bay in our bloodstream. However, in allergic people the bloodstream has programmed white cells to attack surfaces of particles that are not viruses or bacteria, and may be substances with which we come into contact all the time. And the body doesn't have to meet the substances just in the blood: cells known as mast cells that lie in the surface of the lung passages and airsacs, and through the digestive system, are "scouts" for the army of white blood cells. If the allergen meets a mast cell a signal is sent to call reinforcements, and inflammation results.

The mast cells do more than this, though, as they also release their own weapons on the allergen particle when it hits: a mixture of chemicals of which the most potent is histamine. Histamine causes the production of more mucus, and sets off local inflammation of the area.

Remembering the example of the sprained ankle, you know that an inflamed part of the body remains swollen for some time. This is because the white blood cells don't just disperse as quickly as they arrived. They stay in the area and only gradually, over some days, does the swelling subside. This is true of allergic asthma. After an attack the air passages remain inflamed for some days, and recovery is slow.

Nonallergic Asthma

When asthma is caused by something that does not cause inflammation, only bronchial spasm, it is called nonallergic asthma. Asthma produced by cold air or a humidity change is nonallergic asthma.

Some people have asthmatic reactions to tobacco smoke, strong perfumes or smoke from fires. If they are tested they are not allergic to the tobacco particles or wood ash, but nevertheless the body reacts to them by going into bronchial spasm.

Sometimes this reaction is called twitchy airways, or irritable airways. Whatever its name, it can result in asthma just as surely as allergic asthma. However, because there is no inflammation of the air passages, when the irritant disappears recovery is much quicker than after an allergic attack.

It is not clear why some people have nonallergic asthma reactions to substances most of the population finds harmless.

Triggers

Asthma triggers are diverse and are generally categorized as follows.

- **Specific, atopic, allergic irritants:** seasonal pollens and molds and all-year-round occurring substances which include house dust mites, animals and certain foods.
- **Nonspecific, nonallergic irritants:** such as exercise, emotions, atmosphere, pollution, chemicals, food additives and infection.

Allergic Triggers

Allergic triggers are often very small particles: small enough to be mistaken by the body for viruses or bacteria (which are not as large as human cells).

DUST MITES
The most common allergic trigger is dust mite populations. The mite is too tiny to be seen, but it is still too large for the human body to have an allergic reaction to it. Its droppings, however, are light enough to float into the air and be inhaled, and it is these that set off the allergic reaction. It is estimated that up to 75 per cent of all asthmatics may be allergic to the dust mite.

Despite its name, the dust mite does not live in dust, but loves furnishings such as mattresses, carpets, cushions, pillows and quilts. If you are susceptible to dust mite, be wary of sitting for long times on old couches: these can be dust mite havens. Populations of millions can live in a mattress and many asthmatics find their asthma is worst at night. The mite eats the wastes from our bodies: the tiny particles of skin, for example, that we constantly shed.

To combat dust mites you should minimize the places where they can live. Protective covers can be bought that completely enclose mattresses, and nonallergenic pillows are available that are not good homes for mites. Down comforters and quilts are also dust mite paradises. Mites are killed by temperatures higher than 130°F (and by freezing), so wash whatever you can in temperatures above this or use hot-air dryers. Vacuuming with ordinary vacuum cleaners does not get rid of mites, though vacuuming a mattress regularly will cut down on their food supply, and thus prevent a population explosion. Some sufferers may find that wearing a face mask while vacuuming helps prevent attacks.

Carpets are comfortable on the feet, and can be treated with chemicals that will kill mites living in them, but vacuuming does not pick up mites very successfully from carpet. An alternative is to have wooden, tiled or linoleum floors throughout the house (especially the bedrooms), which do not harbor mites.

Dust mites need reasonable humidity in order to survive and many asthmatics find their asthma improves when they vacation in mountainous areas. This is because high mountain air is very dry and the dust mite population is consequently very low. Equally, in cold climates asthmatics may find their condition improves during winter as the dust mite population is killed by icy temperatures.

POLLEN
Pollen is a major allergen. Recent Australian research has shown, in fact, that it is not the pollen grains themselves that are causing asthma, but the combination of pollen grains and water. When wet, the pollen grain breaks open and releases even tinier particles that reach the air passages, and it is these that aggravate asthma. In dry weather the whole grain is more likely to be caught in the upper respiratory tract, the nose and throat, and cause hay fever instead of asthma.

Asthmatics will know that not all plant species release pollen that causes problems. Plants that are wind-pollinated generally produce a huge amount of tiny pollen grains, while insect-pollinated plants release much fewer, larger grains that do not float in the air in the same way. It is the former that trigger asthma. Pollen-related asthma is often seasonal, coinciding with flowering time. If you live in the country there is not a lot you can do to minimize your exposure to pollens at certain times of the year, but here are a few tips to help you to reduce the pollens in a suburban garden.

- Pave areas instead of having lawns.
- If you have lawns make sure they are mown low and flowerheads never have the chance to form.
- Plant insect-pollinated plants instead of wind-pollinated ones. Wind-pollinated species shed their light pollen into the air in enormous quantities, while the heavier, insect-pollinated types are much less likely to be allergic triggers.
- Be wary of plants with heavy fragrance: these can also trigger asthma.

ANIMALS

Although people may say they are allergic to cats, horses or birds, in fact they are allergic to "dander," the tiny particles of skin and hair that the animal sheds constantly. Even entering a house where a cat has been in the past can give susceptible people an asthma attack. Avoiding that particular type of animal is really the only solution for such asthmatics.

OTHER ALLERGENS

Of course, there are many other allergens that cause asthma. A by no means complete list would include fur, feathers, wool, perfumes, chemicals used in hair care products and cosmetics, insecticides, household cleaners and disinfectants, oil and gasoline fumes, and the fumes from gas heaters. Three of the most common are molds, foods and drugs.

Mold spores are being increasingly suspected as causes of asthma because, like pollen, they can be released into the air in huge numbers. You don't have to live in a damp suburb to have mold in your home, either: molds can survive in a variety of places. Badly ventilated cupboards, bathroom corners, kitchen bins or even drawers and wardrobes can harbor them. Never put clothes away damp and don't have overwatered houseplants to brighten up your rooms. Many bathroom cleaners now contain ingredients that kill molds.

Some people are allergic to specific foods and will develop asthma whenever they eat them. The most common allergens in our diet are dairy products, yeast products (bread, beer), eggs, chocolate and a number of food additives, particularly preservatives, colorings and monosodium glutamate.

Finally, drugs can cause asthma attacks in sensitive people. The types of drugs that have been implicated in these reactions are aspirin, nonsteroidal anti-inflammatory drugs (NSAIDs) and beta-blockers.

Aspirin is found as an ingredient of many brands of cold and flu medications, and asthmatics should be careful to check the ingredients when buying them. A relative of aspirin, a salicylate, is found in some foods, and this can also affect sensitive people.

NSAIDs are anti-inflammatory medications that are often prescribed for back pain, joint pain, swelling resulting from arthritis and gout. Beta-blockers are usually given to stabilize irregular heartbeat, or to relieve angina.

Nonallergic Triggers

Nonallergic triggers can be physical or emotional, as diverse as a strong scent and a family argument. Triggers are usually specific to the person, though, so it is necessary for the asthmatic to recognize what causes his or her asthma and avoid it.

Tobacco smoke is a particularly well-known trigger, and anyone with asthma should attempt to live in as smoke-free an atmosphere as possible. Chemicals that cause asthma are often those with a strong smell: paints and solvents can set off an attack as well as perfume. Smog (the pollution produced by engines and factories that hangs around in the atmosphere because of prevailing weather instead of dispersing as usual) is a danger to asthmatics, and smog-alert days are declared when the level of pollution in the atmosphere is likely to reach a point that it will trigger asthma or bronchial attacks.

Asthmatics may also be badly affected by all kinds of emotional stresses: laughing and crying can bring on attacks, as can arguments, family upheavals, or excessive pressure as a result of school or university examinations.

Physical stress is well known as a trigger for asthma and many asthmatics will start to wheeze after only short exercise. This does not mean that people with asthma should not exercise, for health is dependent on fitness. The asthmatic should choose a sport or pastime that does not induce asthma, generally one that does not require bursts of activity and the resultant taking in of deep breaths of air. Asthma-inducing sports involve the quick inspiration of unusually large amounts of cold or dry air; the bronchioles do not have time to humidify or warm this air, and this is what is believed to cause the problem. Swimming is an ideal exercise for asthmatics (see Chapter 7).

Many asthmatics find that the weather has an effect on their asthma. Some people find that cold weather triggers attacks, while for others high humidity or thunderstorms are more dangerous. It may be that some types of weather are connected with high levels of particular allergens – pollutants on a still day or pollen on a windy one, for instance – but most weather-induced bronchial spasms are probably caused by the asthmatic's airways having difficulty responding to the temperature or humidity.

Finally, physical stresses due to your body being injured or out of proper alignment may be a contributing factor in asthma. If your spinal column is misaligned your entire upper body can be under pressure, and you may be predisposed to asthma of the bronchial spasm variety. Equally, if you are under extreme nervous tension your lungs are more likely to react badly to an irritant and set off an asthma attack.

It will be clear that asthma attacks can occur very suddenly, without any warning, if an asthmatic meets a potent trigger in his or her surroundings. It is also true that asthma due to an allergic response can build up for hours or days, the inflammation gradually getting worse and the condition only becoming apparent when the attack is well under way. Using a peak flow meter will help give warning of slow deterioration, but asthmatics must always be on guard for an attack out of the blue.

Occupational Asthma

Exposure to offending allergen or irritant substances in the workplace puts many asthma-sensitive people at great risk. Certain occupations and particular industries have been associated with high levels of occupational asthma. These include the heavy metal and chemical industries as well as bakeries and supermarkets. Housepainters are at risk because of chemicals in the paints, as are hairdressers who are exposed to chemicals in colorings and gas station attendants surrounded by fuel fumes. Hobbies that utilize chemicals, such as photography, painting and gardening, can also be unsafe for the asthma sufferer.

Asthma flares can occur immediately on exposure to an offending substance or reactions may be delayed until evening. A telltale sign of occupational asthma is that symptoms fade over the weekend or during holidays.

It can take weeks, months or years before workplace-caused asthma becomes evident. Grain dust, for instance, can be carried spasmodically by the wind from nearby flour mills to a workplace and the allergy may only develop over a period of time.

Cigarette smokers are much more likely to develop occupational asthma than nonsmokers. This is because the linings of the air passages are damaged by cigarette smoke and they then react more to other triggers.

It is important to understand there is a risk that long-term occupational asthma can lead to serious and irreversible airway obstruction. If occupational asthma has been diagnosed, it is best to change your workplace; if you can't do this, at least try to avoid the offending irritant. If these options are not possible you could wear a face mask or use medications before exposure.

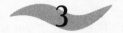

LIVING WITH
ASTHMA

So you have been diagnosed as having asthma and have had an asthma attack. What can you expect? A lifetime of taking drugs, frequent trips to your health practitioner and occasional visits to the hospital? This may be the case, but you might be able to reduce your reliance on medication by taking some practical steps.

All the research, drugs and professional health care available today have not improved society's overall state of health or halted the rising incidence of asthma. Our hospital lines are longer, doctors' waiting rooms are fuller and people seem less healthy than they used to be, although some are living longer.

The most intelligent thing we can do is to know and understand our own body. Good health is an efficiently functioning body. Good health is reflected in a happy and a joyous attitude toward living. Unfortunately most people place their health in the hands of others when, in fact, our health is our own responsibility.

People with asthma **can** do something to improve their health. We can all take charge of our lifestyle; we **can** nurture and nourish our body to perform at its best.

Recognizing Danger Signals

Asthma is a variable illness requiring daily assessment and self-management. As you recognize the nature and symptoms of your asthma you will learn to adapt your lifestyle to reduce exposure to your specific triggers. Constant awareness of your condition will become a way of life for you.

Even a mild attack can escalate quickly and normal breathing may deteriorate rapidly into a dreaded "choking and gasping for air" phase. It is imperative that any attack should not get out of control. You must be aware of your "normal" breathing pattern and your "attack" mode of breathing, so that when your breathing deteriorates seriously, you get help immediately.

There are some very real danger signals that an attack is out of control and medical assistance is needed without delay.

- Breathing is short and gasping.
- Wheezing ceases, which means so little air is going into your airways that the chest has been silenced.
- You can't get up from a bed or chair without difficulty.
- You are sweating profusely, feel feverish, and are weak and trembling.
- You can only speak a few words between gasps.
- Your lips, tongue or fingernails become blue. This final symptom is an EMERGENCY signal of sinking into unconsciousness. An ambulance and doctor must be called immediately.

Not all asthmatics have such obvious signs of an acute attack. There are many people whose breathing deteriorates very slowly over a long time, sometimes days or weeks, and who do not have noticeable wheezes. The only immediate symptom of an acute attack in such an asthmatic may be muddled conversation or behavior (a sign that the brain is not getting sufficient oxygen) or a loss of color in the face, with a gray–blue tinge appearing around the nose and mouth. Although all asthmatics should monitor their lung capacity regularly, it is vitally important that those with "invisible" symptoms should be extra vigilant in doing so. A peak flow meter is the most convenient way to do this at home (see pages 25–6).

Monitoring Your Asthma

The best way to take control of your health is to understand your condition and how it may fluctuate from day to day. As asthma can vary dramatically from one person to another, and may produce a wide range of symptoms, individualized assessment by a medical practitioner is your first priority. It may be that a visit to a respiratory specialist will be necessary while your asthma is being investigated.

When your asthma has been clearly defined – and allied respiratory conditions identified or dismissed – you should continue to be closely monitored by a medical practitioner. Consult the same doctor regularly so that he or she becomes familiar with your health. It is important that you develop a partnership with your doctor so that you are working together towards the same goal. You cannot successfully control your asthma if you are not being assessed accurately, so if you are not happy with the attention you are receiving, change your doctor and find one who will give you the support and management plan you need.

There is nothing more frightening than an asthma attack. An attack must be prevented if warning signs appear, and prescribed medication taken to stop it. In the event of a severe attack everything possible must be done to ensure the asthma is controlled, as an untreated attack may lead to death. Hospitalization may be necessary, and common sense should guide you about when emergency care should be sought.

We do not intend you to use the complementary concepts outlined in this book when an asthma attack is severe. For instance, when asthma's restricted breathing has developed it is difficult to adopt the Controlled Pattern Breathing we describe later (see Chapter 6). The breathing exercises are practiced only when you are feeling well and are basically free of asthma. However, we firmly believed that the therapies outlined in Part Two of this book, and Controlled Pattern Breathing in particular, will help lessen your asthma, improve your health and ultimately reduce your reliance on medication.

Prevention is the keynote of all these complementary concepts and you should investigate and adopt those most suited to your particular condition and of the most benefit to you. None of the alternative therapies should be viewed as the sole means of managing your asthma. Discuss your selection with your medical practitioner and always ensure that you are both happy about the most appropriate asthma care for you.

Peak Flow Meters

A peak flow meter gives a quick, reliable lung-capacity measurement in liters per minute or seconds. Obtainable fairly inexpensively from most pharmacies, a peak flow meter enables you to keep a daily check and maintain records of your asthma levels. A graph of these readings will establish if and when you are at your best, the variability of your condition, and whether a change of treatment, or your response to medication during an attack, has been effective. You will be able to assess the degree to which your airways are affected before and after physical activity and what progress you make over a period of time.

Using a peak flow meter.

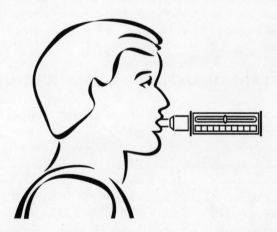

The severity of your condition determines how frequently you need to use a peak flow meter. Some may have to record their peak flow three times a day, but those with mild asthma need only take readings when symptoms are evident, for example

----

during the pollen season or when exposed to allergens. Very little time is needed to take a reading and record it on a chart.

The sample chart below shows the variation that can occur over a few weeks.

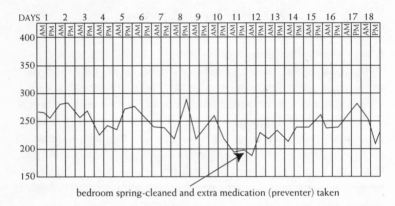

bedroom spring-cleaned and extra medication (preventer) taken

Peak flow chart of a 10-year-old boy.

Information on the specific use of peak flow meters is supplied with each instrument and your medical practitioner will advise you how frequently you should monitor your asthma with it.

Taking Orthodox Medication

Most asthmatics carry an inhaler or a spray to help relieve an attack. Some may not have had an attack for many years, but still take their puffer "just in case." They need the psychological crutch of knowing that immediate relief is at hand.

And attacks can appear without warning. Going on vacation or changing your habits temporarily can bring you in contact with allergens, or just create stress, and may precipitate an attack requiring treatment. When asthma medication is inhaled it travels straight to the irritated air passages and eases the distress. However, the principles and techniques suggested in Part Two of this book are designed to do what medication does in preventing asthma or relieving a mild attack.

That does not mean an asthmatic should not take prescribed medication. In fact orthodox medication may be essential if you are to reach a state of health where your asthma will respond to complementary therapies, and in any acute attack prescribed medication **must** be taken promptly.

Orthodox medicine used in the treatment of asthma is classified in four categories.

1 **Relievers** or **bronchodilators** counter the
   bronchospasms and help open up the air passages that
   contract during attacks. Various kinds of drugs act as
   bronchodilators – adrenalin, salbutamol, terbutaline and
   theophyllines being four – and some of the most
   commonly prescribed inhalers are albuterol sulfate
   (Ventolin and Proventil).
2 **Protectors** do the same job as relievers but keep the
   airways open for a longer period than the above group
   of bronchodilators. They are usually taken on a regular
   basis when bronchodilators are not sufficiently effective.
   Serevent is one commonly prescribed brand.
3 **Preventers** do not relax the airway muscles and reverse
   an attack, but instead decrease the inflammation in the
   air passages over a much longer period of time. They
   are very helpful in controlling chronic asthma. They are
   taken daily whether or not you are suffering from an
   asthma attack.
      There are two kinds of preventive medications:
   steroid and non-steroid. The steroids, such as
   beclomethasone dipropionate(Vanceril) are taken in
   such small doses that they do not have major side-
   effects. Non-steroid inhalations, such as with cromolyn
   sodium (Intal), also do not reverse airway muscle spasm,
   but if taken before exposure to an allergen can prevent
   symptoms.
4 **Acute savers** are only used in a very severe attack and
   for a short time: a week or so. These include oral
   steroids at high dosage and high doses of bronchodilators.

In an emergency, such as when an asthmatic is admitted to the hospital, adrenalin may be administered. Adrenalin relieves a very severe bout of asthma in a short space of time. However use of adrenalin must be closely monitored by a medical practitioner, in conjunction with a strict asthma management plan.

METHODS OF TAKING MEDICATION

Medication can be administered through an inhaler, a spacer or nebulizer; taken as a tablet or in syrup form.

The most common inhalers are the metered-dose, pressurized inhalers that spray the medication, plus a propellant, into the back of the throat. Many people do not use these inhalers correctly and it has been found that more medication reaches the lungs of asthmatics if a spacer is attached to the inhaler.

More environmentally friendly inhalers, such as the Turbuhaler and Rotahaler, are now on the market; these dispense a dry powder. They are propellant-free and are less likely to cause irritation and coughing when the medication is taken. The low pressure needed to activate the Turbuhaler means that children as young as 18 months can be taught to use it effectively.

When asthma is severe a nebulizer may be recommended. A nebulizer ensures that even more medication reaches the lungs than does a spacer. The medication is put into the nebulizer in solution and an air pump delivers it to the mouth and nose, via a mask, as a very fine spray under pressure.

There are side effects, however slight, associated with any medication, and you should ask your medical practitioner exactly what these may be when you are prescribed a new drug. Consider these effects in relation to yourself and be aware if these contraindications appear. You should report any side effects promptly to your doctor. Recent research indicates that people who **overuse** bronchodilators may in fact be damaging their lungs, so puffers should only be used to relieve symptoms.

However, it is most important to prevent an asthma attack taking place. Until you have mastered the techniques of Controlled Pattern Breathing in Part Two, and relaxation, you should take medication at the first hint of any attack.

ASTHMA IN CHILDREN

The first asthma attack a child has is often a frightening experience for both child and parents. Suddenly the family can be awakened in the middle of the night by a child who complains he or she cannot breathe. The family finds itself in the emergency room of the local hospital, where the child has a mask put over his or her face. It's all very strange and upsetting.

The diagnosis of asthma in children isn't always like this, of course. Sometimes parents tell the doctor that the child has a persistent night time cough following a cold virus, and are surprised when the doctor's response is "Asthma."

So what can you expect if your child is an asthmatic? Asthma in children can be mild or severe, and attacks can be rare or frequent. Some children may find themselves in the hospital at frequent intervals, while others may never need anything more than an occasional visit to the doctor for a checkup.

It is true, too, that many children will grow out of it: although in some parts of the world one in four children is now diagnosed as asthmatic to some degree, by the time they are teenagers this has dropped to one in seven, and 80 per cent of asthmatic children will be free of any symptoms

----

when they are adults. Boys are more likely to be asthmatics than girls, for reasons as yet unknown.

Since asthma can be a life-threatening condition, it is vital that parents monitor their children and ensure that all necessary medication is taken. It is much easier to prevent an attack beginning than to treat a full-blown one, and parents should be aware that children are often slow to recognize the signs of asthma in themselves. If your child has asthma it is necessary for you, the parent, to be vigilant on his or her behalf.

Preventing an asthma attack in your children isn't just a matter of making sure they are taking their medication, though. Asthma is often triggered by allergens in the environment, for instance, and there is much that can be done by careful planning around the home to reduce the incidence and severity of attacks. Equally important is encouraging your child to practice techniques and exercises that will improve the condition. Finally, parents may like to introduce their children to some alternative therapies to see if they respond; we have indicated in Part Two of this book if any therapy is not suitable for children.

Will My Child Develop Asthma?

If you or your partner is asthmatic you may worry that your child is likely to be asthmatic also. There are as yet no tests that can be done to check whether any particular child is likely to develop asthma (although research is currently trying to discover exactly which genes and chromosomes are linked to the incidence of asthma, and a test may be possible in the future), but it is agreed that asthma runs in families. Asthma is also linked to allergies: families with histories of allergies are likely to have asthmatic members, and asthma and eczema are commonly found together.

Even though your family may carry the genes for asthma it does not necessarily mean your child will have asthma. The child may have a predisposition to it, but asthma will not appear unless it is triggered in some way, and parents can minimize the chance of their child developing asthma by ensuring the child avoids potential triggers.

Research has shown conclusively that children who are

breastfed exclusively for the first six months of life are less likely to develop asthma. It also appears that if you can keep the potential allergens a baby is exposed to at a minimum (again, the first six months of life seem to be the crucial time) then asthma may be avoided or only appear mildly. This means keeping dust mites down and not introducing pets into the household **before** you suspect your child has asthma. Most importantly, if anyone in the house smokes, they should give it up. There is conclusive evidence that asthma rates are higher among children brought up in homes with parents who smoke.

Asthma Triggers

The recommendations in Chapter 2, "Living with Asthma," for minimizing exposure to triggers, are also applicable to children, but there are some extra precautions you might like to try.

DUST MITES
Dust mites are a major trigger of asthma. They live in bedding, carpets, soft toys – all things that new parents fill a baby's room with. Dust mites are killed by temperatures above 130°F, or by freezing, so make sure that all soft toys and bedding are regularly washed on a hot cycle, or frozen if they are not suitable for washing. Hot-air dryers operate at a sufficient heat to kill the mites. Some parents have two identical soft toys on rotation, so that the child does not miss one when it is in the wash.

Recommendations for bedding are the same as for adults: use nonallergenic pillows and avoid feather-filled quilts. Ensure the mattress is vacuumed regularly and is dry, as dust mites love damp habitats. You can envelop a mattress in a plastic protector.

Carpets are comfortable for small feet, but many parents of asthmatic children find it preferable to have wooden or linoleum floors in their bedrooms that do not harbor mites, as vacuuming is not very successful at picking up the mites. Carpets can also be treated with chemicals or tannic acid that kill the mites. Blinds are more practical than curtains for an asthmatic child's bedroom, but if you choose curtains make sure you wash them regularly, not just once a year.

PETS

Pet dander, the small particles of skin and hair shed by cats and dogs, is a known asthma trigger. If you already have a much loved pet, though, it can be impossible to make the decision to part with it because of the **possibility** the baby-to-come may be allergic to it. However, don't introduce a new pet into the household while a child is very small, and never let a pet get into the habit of sleeping in a child's room or on his or her bed.

Some children have asthmatic reactions to horses, mice, rabbits or guinea pigs also.

DIET

As mentioned above, there is evidence that babies at risk of developing asthma are benefited by being breastfed for at least six months. You should also be careful when introducing solid foods into the diet. Dairy foods of all kinds are often allergic triggers, and wheat-based foods affect some people. Oranges, strawberries, eggs, nuts ... the list goes on. However, you can't – and should not attempt to – eliminate every potential allergen from your child's diet. Just be observant, and if the child shows any ill effects or possible allergy after eating a new food, be wary about making it a permanent part of the diet.

Warning Signs

How can you tell if your child is having a bad asthma attack, especially if the child is too small to be able to understand what is happening or communicate with you properly? Asthma isn't always immediately noticeable – it creeps up slowly, then suddenly you realize your child is having difficulty breathing. There are some signs you should be alert to at all times, as they are indications that the child may be struggling with reduced lung capacity.

- Persistent coughing at night, although there is no particular sign of a cold or cough during the day.
- Unusual breathlessness or coughing following exercise.
- Lack of appetite.
- Wheeziness.

- Unusual lethargy.
- Unusual itching.
- Loss of color from the face: some children get a "pinched" look around the mouth and nose, and the skin becomes rather gray instead of a healthy pink. If the skin actually looks blue around this area the attack may already be severe and you must take **emergency** action to prevent it getting worse – call medical assistance or an ambulance.

There may, of course, be more obvious signs: the child's breathing may become gradually more and more shallow, the wheeze may become louder and the child may complain of tightness or pain in the chest and difficulty breathing.

What to Do

The most important thing is not to panic. The asthma will become worse if the child is upset or frightened. Do whatever you can to help the child relax: cuddles, soothing music, warm surroundings, comfortable clothes and, naturally, give medication if you have any prescribed.

If the child is suffering from his or her first asthma attack you won't have any preparations made, or medication available. Take the child to a doctor as quickly as possible so that he or she can be assessed immediately and medication given if necessary. If it is the middle of the night and the child is apparently fighting for breath, don't wait until morning – go to an emergency facility immediately.

Remember, sudden breathlessness in the middle of the night is not necessarily asthma. Croup is always a possibility in infants. Croup usually precedes a respiratory infection, and the symptoms sound alarming: a curious barking, gasping, wheezing fight for breath that is generally made worse by the child's terror. Croup symptoms can often be relieved by putting the child in an atmosphere of high humidity. Take the child into the bathroom, close the door and turn on the hot taps. The steam in the atmosphere will loosen the airways and the child will begin to be able to breathe normally again. If breathing does not improve rapidly, however, take the child to the hospital, where they can administer an adrenalin injection that will expand the airways.

Once at the hospital, a baby or small child with breathing problems is always looked after immediately – there's no long wait. If the diagnosis is asthma you will find that a mask is put over the child's face and they will inhale a vaporized medication for a period of time. The emergency procedures themselves may seem frightening to the child, though, as strange doctors and nurses cluster around, machines are wheeled about, tests are done, and sometimes oxygen tanks or drips need to be brought into use and injections given. Parents must keep the child as calm as possible, as panic will only make the struggle for breath worse.

Although the asthma may seem to improve after treatment it is unlikely the child will be immediately discharged, as monitoring needs to be done for a few hours and medication repeated at intervals. It is more likely you will find yourself spending the night in the children's ward. If your child has bad asthma you should be prepared for this: remember to grab a favorite teddy or doll, or their comfort blanket, to take with you to the hospital. A baby who always sleeps with a pacifier will need one in a strange place. Most hospitals make arrangements for parents to stay beside the bed of small children, but this may involve sleeping in a chair or on a hard floor, and you will want a hairbrush and toilet kit in the morning to help freshen up.

After your child has been diagnosed as having asthma, he or she will generally be prescribed medication (often to prevent further bouts as well as to relieve acute attacks) and you should ensure the child takes it as recommended. Discuss with your doctor what you can do to improve the child's health and minimize the drugs needed. Never stop giving the child the prescribed medication without the full agreement of your doctor.

Managing Asthma

Once your child's asthma diagnosis is confirmed you will have to decide how to manage the condition. Your child should have an asthma management plan worked out with your doctor. If you are uncertain about the extent of your child's asthma and how to monitor it, get the child to use a peak flow meter regularly, and then you will know when the asthma is worsening.

If a child is very small it is not possible to introduce them to special breathing techniques or exercises: for such techniques to be useful the child must first understand what he or she is supposed to do. As soon as the child can follow instructions with understanding you should begin the exercises we explain on pages 67–8. Children under five cannot generally perform these exercises satisfactorily, but they can practice blowing up balloons and play blowing games that help them breathe correctly. We describe a number of these games also.

There are other activities that can be extremely beneficial to children suffering from asthma. In particular, you should encourage your child to swim well, as the breathing discipline needed to exhale under water is ideal for asthmatics. (Don't let your child get away with trying to keep his or her head out of the water as they swim: the point of the exercise is to exhale slowly and regularly, as happens during correct breathing for swimming.)

Floating is also excellent for asthmatic children, as it teaches them what to do with their mind and body when a parent asks them to relax. Learning to relax is important, as a relaxed child will breathe more easily. Relaxation has to be learned, though, as it is not a natural state for a child: parents generally know that although a child may be relaxed when asleep, while awake most children do not know **how** to relax. That's why floating is a good idea, as it is impossible to float when one is tense – the body must be completely relaxed to float successfully.

For babies and young infants relaxation cannot be taught, but it is possible for a parent to help them relax by massage, and a relaxed baby will breathe more easily than a tense one. Infant care clinics will often refer you to trained infant massage therapists. Massage may also help relieve colicky or fretful babies.

Relaxation can also be mastered by children through playing games like the elephant walk (see Chapter 6). And, of course, sometimes just a simple cuddle of a baby or child will be reassuring and comforting enough to relieve the child's distress.

Other activities that will help children with asthma control their breathing from the diaphragm are learning to sing or play a wind or brass instrument. Encourage your child to join the school choir or band and choose an instrument within the child's capabilities, physically and musically!

HOME

Take precautions around the house, and particularly in your child's bedroom, as outlined on pages 16–20. Some pamphlets that are printed to give advice to parents suggest no soft toys or books should be allowed in a bedroom, as these accumulate dust so readily. Remember that your house should be a home, not a hospital, and be careful you do not make your child miserable by following such recommendations too zealously: you can't easily take away a teddy that has been the constant companion of a toddler just because of an asthma attack when he is three – this is the time when your child will most need to cuddle it! Freeze it or wash it in hot water regularly instead.

If you suspect your child's asthma may be diet-related, keep a diary of what he or she eats – and make sure you know of any treats they might have eaten at a friend's house or at school. Try to match the asthma pattern with a particular food. If the child's asthma is triggered by a food additive this may be difficult, but it is possible to narrow down the foods that seem to trigger an attack.

One of the most common additives to cause asthmatic reactions is the yellow dye used as a food coloring, tartrazine. Other troublesome additives are sodium metabisulphite and potassium metabisulphite, which are preservatives used in making sausages, dried fruit such as raisins and currants, some fruit yogurts, jams and flavorings. If you suspect an additive is responsible for the asthma, you will have to become adept at reading labels before you buy. Allergy testing may help you pin down exactly what the child is reacting to. (See also "Food Allergies and Additives" in Chapter 8.)

SCHOOL AND CHILDCARE

It is important that the day care center, kindergarten or school knows that your child is an asthmatic, and what medication he or she may need. Child care centers and schools will ask for details of asthma when your child enrolls, and make sure you give all relevant information. If your child is prescribed two medications (one for prevention and one to be taken in the event of an attack), give the school or center clear instructions for their use. Ensure that if it is necessary medication is kept at school; find out where the school stores it, and ask that they take it on outings to swimming pools, playgrounds, etc., where it may most be needed!

Finally, don't feel that your child will be unable to take part in sports because he or she is asthmatic. Many professional sportsmen and women are asthmatics. The physical education teacher should be aware that the child has asthma, and be able to recognize warning signs that might mean he or she is in difficulties and therefore needs assistance; however, with supervision asthmatic children should be able to take their place in all the usual school sporting activities.

VACATIONS

Taking a vacation with an asthmatic child does require a little more planning than usual. You must take into account the likelihood of the child meeting asthma triggers while away: don't plan a vacation on a farm in spring and summer if you have a child whose asthma is aggravated by pollens. Although sea air is frequently considered good for people with asthma, beware of beach houses with aging mattresses that are a haven for dust mites. Finally, before you go make sure there is sufficient medication – and that the child has actually packed it!

Even the shortest stay away from home needs consideration. If your child is asked to spend the night sleeping over at a friend's house, warn the parents of the asthmatic condition and ensure your child takes medication along – there may be a cat or dog in the house that will trigger an unexpected attack.

Medication for Children

In general, the medication prescribed for children with asthma is much the same as for adults, and information about it is given in Chapter 3. Some powerful drugs that are only used in extreme cases do have side effects, though: certain steroids can affect a child's growth, but are generally not used at anything like sufficient dosage to cause a problem. However, if your child is on steroids and does not appear to be growing at a normal rate, talk this over with your doctor.

The best way of delivering asthma medication is through

the lungs, which is why doctors prescribe inhalers of various kinds for children. The design of these is evolving and they are now easier for children to use correctly than they used to be. Turbuhalers and Rotahalers are particularly suitable for children.

Babies and toddlers can't use inhalers themselves, but they can be given drugs through a spacer, where a mask is put over their face and the parent introduces the vapor at the other end. An alternative is to give infants syrup containing drugs. Although easy to give to a small child, the syrup has two disadvantages: it is slower to act, having to work through the stomach into the bloodstream before it is of use, and it has to be given in larger quantities than the inhaled drugs.

Alternative Treatments for Children

Not all the alternative treatments that we discuss in Part Two of this book will be suitable for children – for instance, a very strict food diet would not be appropriate for a young child. However many, such as homeopathy, Bach flower remedies, vitamins and minerals, and massage, can be of great benefit. There are complementary remedies, in particular homeopathic and herbal remedies, prepared in appropriate doses for asthmatic babies.

Where a particular treatment or technique in Part Two is unsuitable for children to try this is indicated at the beginning of the section describing it.

PART TWO

CONTROLLING
ASTHMA IN
ALTERNATIVE WAYS

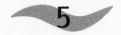

5

ALTERNATIVE
APPROACHES

Our society tends to rely on "pressing a button" to satisfy all our wants. We expect immediate entertainment – press the television or video remote button and there it is; if we need to relax, we have a quick drink; if we feel under pressure, we have a cigarette; if we have a headache, we take a pill; and so on. If we have asthma, it is all too easy just to use the puffer, and rely completely on medication for a quick fix.

Our expectations are that if something is wrong with us, there is a drug or medication to give us immediate relief, or an operation available where and when we want it. It is generally considered that when a problem exists, an immediate answer will be available. Unfortunately life, and health, are not like that. Good health, like a good marriage, needs commitment. We need to be responsible for our own health and not necessarily reliant on medication.

It is an unfortunate fact today that, in Western societies, the number of pills, potions and prescriptions being dispensed is spiralling every year as orthodox practitioners worry about being sued for medical malpractice if they do not prescribe something – anything – when a patient visits them. The result is a lot of buttons being pressed!

It is also true that asthmatics often rely heavily on their spray or puffer, using it as a psychological crutch rather than as a non-preferred treatment. It is not the use of medication which causes concern, but over-reliance on this form of treatment.

There is now a growing body of evidence which suggests that constant dosing with bronchodilators may not be altogether harmless. A study in Dunedin, New Zealand, examined whether using a bronchodilator four times a day improved asthma, made no difference or made it worse. The researchers concluded that it made the underlying condition worse. (Despite these findings, you should not change your medication or dosage without consulting your practitioner.)

Asthmatics, like the rest of society, are tending to rely more and more on medication and are overlooking the importance of other, natural methods to control their condition – methods which may require more time, thought and effort than simply taking medication.

The more you become aware of your own body, and respond to its needs, the more probable it is that you will experience better health. An asthmatic's body will find it difficult to heal if it is being continuously abused with poor diet, excessive medication, lack of exercise, negative thoughts and inadequate rest. All of these stress the body, leading to a depressed immune and healing system. The alternative is to cultivate a fortified immune system and active lifestyle, which will help protect you from the rigors of asthma.

Remember that **you alone** are responsible for your health. So **you** must take steps to understand your body, its functions and needs, and tread the path to "wellness." This is especially so for an asthmatic, because it will take time, perseverance, effort and commitment for you to be successful in gaining relief from your condition. Health has to be worked on and, like most things in life, good health doesn't come easily.

Just as there are 101 reasons for an asthma attack, there are also 101 ways an asthma attack can be avoided. Many alternative techniques can help you reduce your reliance on orthodox medication, and you should seek out practical help to find the complementary techniques that improve your asthma. It has been said that a natural therapist should be the first port of call rather than the last, which is more often the case.

Nevertheless, the lifesaving treatments offered by orthodox medication cannot be underestimated and it would be foolish indeed to reject the use of effective drugs altogether. The alternative treatments described in this book are complements to orthodox medication, not substitutes. Prescribed medication must be taken for immediate relief and to stop an attack. The aim of alternative and natural therapies is to control and, if possible, prevent asthma.

The chapters which follow, in Part Two of this book, offer an eclectic collection of alternative therapies to help asthmatics ease their distress. The most important of these, we believe, is Controlled Pattern Breathing, which is described in Chapter 6. Many other factors have a vital bearing on your asthmatic condition, however, and should not be neglected: regular exercise to ensure physical fitness, and a healthy diet to improve and protect your immune system, are extremely important. Also included are many natural remedies which will improve your body's response to outside factors and asthmatic triggers.

We are not claiming that all the ideas in this section are of equal value to people with asthma. Some of the therapies may only result in greater relaxation – but being relaxed really does prevent asthma attacks from becoming severe. The therapeutic mind and body methods and lifestyle topics offer you various options for broadening your self-help scope, so that you can handle your condition and improve your overall health.

Asthma **can** be prevented, so instead of taking things for granted and believing nothing can be done to alleviate your condition, take up the challenge this book offers and travel the road to an asthma-free, healthy lifestyle!

6

BREATHING IS
LIVING

If we don't breathe we don't live – it's as simple as that. We breathe about 11,375 liters (2500 gallons) of air a day via our nose or mouth, through the larynx and windpipe (trachea), down the bronchial tubes branching from the trachea, through the smaller bronchioles and still smaller tubes in the lungs, finally to the alveoli, the small saclike structures from which oxygen enters the blood.

The oxygen that ultimately reaches the bloodstream has travelled through our body's filter system. Foreign particles in the air can be trapped by mucus in the nasal passages, windpipe, bronchi or bronchioles, and then the hair-like structures called cilia which line these passages help propel this polluted mucus back into the mouth so that it can be discharged. This filtering system, along with sneezing and coughing mechanisms, clears the airways of unwanted particles.

At the same time, the amount of air passing to and from the alveoli and bronchioles is controlled by the expansion and contraction of the bronchioles' smooth muscle walls. Additionally, some respiratory bacteria and viruses can be neutralized by antibody reactions in the airway linings and by cells in the alveoli called macrophages. These defenders protect the integrity of the airways, allowing oxygen to enter.

Breathing Patterns

If we don't breathe correctly we invite ill health. Most people assume that the way they breathe is how everybody breathes – that it happens naturally, so what is there to think about? Well, there is much to think about!

Do you know how your breathing pattern affects your health? And that incorrect breathing habits mean an inadequate oxygen supply is getting to the billions of cells in our body? The good news is that we can change our breathing pattern, improve the supply of oxygen, and thus purify and enrich our blood, adding vitality to our body and our mind.

Our breathing pattern has been with us since birth, so it does take a lot of unlearning. But no matter how old you are, you can learn to breathe correctly.

The majority of people inhale a limited amount of air, and shallow breathing becomes a habit. We have to learn the art of breathing our way to better health. It's easy! The action of the diaphragm, that large muscle separating the lungs from the abdominal cavity, is the key to breathing. When we inhale and inflate the lungs, the diaphragm flattens out. When we exhale and deflate the lungs, it rises. Actually, this is what **should** happen. However, most people only take shallow breaths and do not use their diaphragm properly. Our aim is to improve the activity of the diaphragm, which will increase the intake of oxygen. People with asthma need a greater supply of oxygen than nonasthmatics and can relieve the tension in their respiratory passages by breathing correctly.

How an Asthmatic Breathes

Patients often describe asthma as extreme tightness in the chest and restriction in the throat. Asthmatics tend to breathe shallowly and high up in their upper chest. This short breathing pattern, with limited diaphragm movement, produces two kinds of body development that are not ideal.

Type A usually has a slightly caved-in chest, with limited upper chest development. The body is often bent, with shoulders hunched almost as if they are afraid to breathe.

Type B can be barrel-chested, through habitual overbreathing,

Type A body structure.   Type B body structure.

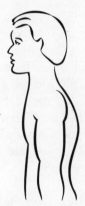 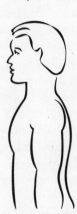

using the upper chest more than they should as they continually try to get enough precious air.

Often the lower torsos of both Types A and B are under-developed because they are not using their diaphragms to help them breathe.

Both types often reject any suggestion of taking exercise to improve their chest and body structure. They have become locked into an emotional circle of thinking that because they can't breathe properly, they can't exercise. But their problem is really a simple lack of physical rhythm, which only needs to be regulated to restore harmonious breathing action in the body.

Learning to correct an unnatural mode of breathing is essential for the relief of asthma. It does require effort, practice and perseverance, and may take some three to four months to master, but you will be doing your body a favor by establishing healthy breathing habits for the rest of your life.

Learning to Relax with Controlled Breathing

Have you ever noticed what happens when someone comes home from a pressure-filled day at work or has just finished an exhausting game or exercise routine? Usually they will sit down in a comfortable chair and let out a long, slow sigh. The muscles ease and the whole body relaxes.

During the day's activities, we often fail to recognize that we are holding ourselves stiff and tight. We grip the steering wheel while driving the car, sit hunched over a desk or grasp a book while reading. How often do you find yourself feeling stressed, anxious, tense? Test yourself occasionally and see if you are clutching that steering wheel or book too tightly. Are you bent over the desk unnecessarily? If you are, then stop what you are doing, let out a long, slow sigh. Repeat a few times and you will feel the difference! You are relaxing. Now you are consciously encouraging yourself to relax by breathing out long, slow and letting go.

The more air you expel from your body, the greater the next air intake will be. Your lungs become hungry for air, which stimulates the automatic impulse to breathe in. Simple, isn't it? So the emphasis should be on breathing **out long and slow** and letting breathing in happen naturally. Breathing **out** long and slow produces a relaxation response. Try it. Notice how your shoulders droop, your head drops towards your chest. You just let go. This wonderful state is the level of relaxation all asthmatics should strive for so that it becomes their normal way of life. **Learning to relax is as important as learning to breathe correctly, and the techniques are dependent on one another for success**.

Practice the following relaxation technique when you are feeling well so that when anxiety or stress overwhelm you, you are equipped with relaxation skills to help you cope. Some asthma attacks are triggered by stress, but all are made worse by anxiety or panic, so learning to relax really does improve asthma.

RELAX AND LET GO

Breathe **out** long, slow; relax and let go.
Breathe **out** long, slow; relax and let go.
Feel the tension fading away, relaxing you more and
more with each long, slow breath **out**, down to the tips
of your fingers and toes.
Let breathing in happen naturally.
Breathe **out** long, slow; relax and let go.

Practice this exercise from time to time and learn to relax. When you feel overwhelmed with worries, and an asthma attack seems imminent, take the time to sit down, perform the relaxation exercise and prevent that attack before it starts.

Controlled Pattern Breathing

Ron's experience is that asthma can be avoided and a normal, breathe-easy existence is within everyone's reach. You only have to learn to breathe correctly.

His underlying principle in controlling asthma is the yin and yang concept of positive and negative attitudes: that everything has an opposite, for instance dark/light, male/female. We can be happy or we can be sad, we can be hot or we can be cold, and we can be in good health or poor health. In all these situations there is an element of choice: we can influence whether we are happy or sad, by being deliberately optimistic or pessimistic; we can take off clothes if we are hot, or put them on if we are cold. The same is true of health: we can influence our health by what we do and our mental attitude. Unhappy or stressed people are frequently in poor health.

Asthmatics also have to consider how they breathe. They have choices. They can breathe air in and out with short gasps or they can breathe in and out long; they can breathe high up in their chests or they can breathe deeply from the diaphragm. Asthmatics' short intake of air, high in the chest, is negative breathing – it is not doing anything to help get oxygen into the body. But if they choose to learn the opposite they will be breathing positively!

Something as simple as breathing can profoundly affect your health. If you restore breathing harmony and balance to your body your asthma will improve, your energy levels will increase and you will be bursting with good health.

Ron is often asked "What do you think is the single most important method for the relief of asthma?" There is no doubt in his mind that while other therapies are extremely helpful, Controlled Pattern Breathing is by far the most useful and everyone with asthma should practice it.

Controlled Pattern Breathing exercises

As explained above, by expelling as much air as possible from your body you are forced to breathe a large amount of air in. The more the body rids itself of the stale carbon dioxide, the greater will be the intake of clean air and oxygen. Once the air is fully expelled from the lungs using the diaphragm, it is natural that the diaphragm will also be used to fill the lungs with air.

Most people use their diaphragm to do about 65 per cent of the breathing work, by making it push against the lungs to exhale and lowering it to inhale. In contrast, the diaphragm of someone with asthma may do as little as 30 per cent. Once diaphragmatic breathing out has been mastered, breathing in deeply using the diaphragm will follow automatically. Controlled Pattern Breathing ensures that the asthmatic breathes using all the lungs – first taking air into the lower lungs using the diaphragm and then into the upper chest using rib cage expansion.

How do you do it? Let's start right now! First, you must be calm and relaxed, so that your body can respond more easily to an altered breathing pattern. If necessary, do the relaxation exercise from page 46 before you begin the Controlled Breathing Pattern.

▶ Stand upright, or sit in a chair, shoulders relaxed but not bent forward, arms hanging loosely, legs slightly bent.

▶ Relax your lips and have them slightly open so that when you breathe out you make a '**puhhhh**' sound, as the air is expelled LONG and SLOW.

▶ Concentrate on breathing **out** as far as you comfortably can. Air hunger will activate the in breath. Don't raise your shoulders. Breathe **out**, LONG and SLOW.

▶ Gradually extend your breathing **out** to 5 seconds or so, with only a short breath in of 1–2 seconds. Don't breathe out so far that you create a wheeze. You shouldn't feel distressed.

Practice for about 5–10 minutes per day. It may take some time for your body to become accustomed to this changed breathing – weeks, even months.

The long-term goal is to be able to breathe out for 30 seconds. There are many times during the day you can practice: when sitting quietly, walking slowly, waiting at traffic lights and, especially, when in bed before going to sleep. Keep remembering to breathe **out** LONG and SLOW. Just let breathing in happen naturally.

You will now have mastered breathing at the right rhythm, but are you using your diaphragm to do it? This is the second step in learning Controlled Pattern Breathing.

CONTROLLING DIAPHRAGM EXERCISE

► Lie or sit comfortably. Place your hands flat on your stomach, with middle fingertips touching, just below your navel.

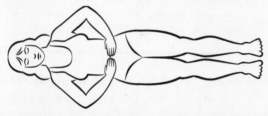

► Slowly and gently breathe **out**, pressing down and in with your fingers to expel as much air as comfortably possible.

► As you allow breathing in to take place naturally, direct the air down towards your diaphragm, making your tummy rise and your fingers part. You will notice your lower chest automatically fills with air.

► Breathe **out** LONG and SLOW, again expelling as much air as possible. Your fingertips will return to their starting position.

► Do not be tempted to overbreathe. Just take it easy and stay within your capacity. Do not allow yourself to reach the point where you are gasping for air. This would only aggravate your condition.

Continue practicing this pattern of breathing for some time and be sure you have mastered it before progressing to the next stage.

Using the long and slow diaphragmatic breathing
explained above:
▶ breathe **out** slowly, PAUSE and hold for a second,
breathe in, PAUSE for a second.

Continue practicing this pattern until you feel comfortable with it.

▶ The final step extends the breathing pattern by
developing a rhythm of breathing **out** to the
count of six, pausing for a second, and in to the
count of three.
▶ The irregular **out**/in count should be varied and
increased, depending on your progress, to the point
that you can breathe **out** for 8–12 seconds and in for
2–4 seconds.

Professional swimmers use this breathing rhythm. They breathe
out under the water for four, five or six strokes and in for one.
Swimming benefits asthma, as does walking, running, cycling and
singing, as long as the breathing technique is used.

TIPS FOR BETTER BREATHING

● Watch a runner in action. Observe their technique of a
short inhalation and a long expiration – a sprinter will
push air out for almost a full 100 meters. The same
breathing pattern can be seen in a football or soccer
player kicking a ball, or a rower pulling on the oars of a
boat. The basic strategy of athletes who wish to take as
much oxygen as possible into their bodies is to consciously
breathe **out** when an effort is involved and breathe in
when the effort is lessened.
● An opera singer breathes out for a long time when
singing – long **out** and short in. Practice
singing ... even if you don't have a good voice –
that doesn't matter if it helps your asthma. Sing while
you are working around the house, especially songs

with lots of words; sing along with the radio. A
vocalist or singer "throws the voice" – breathing **out**
long and in short. There's no harm in trying it, after
all, people who sing or whistle while they are
working are usually happy people – and happy people
are usually healthy people!

• If your asthma is not allergy triggered by the
  dreaded chores of vacuuming, sweeping, lawn
  mowing, window cleaning or painting, but perhaps
  you find yourself breathless through exertion, you
  can make light work of these tasks by using
  Controlled Pattern Breathing.

• You've probably heard the saying: "Laughter is the
  best medicine." It is also a great breathing exercise.
  "Internal jogging" is the way Dr. William Fry, a
  psychiatry professor at Stanford University's School of
  Medicine, described laughing. Laughing involves the
  same muscle activity as exercising. It brings more
  oxygen into the lungs and cells and helps rid the
  body of carbon dioxide. It relaxes you. And, as Dr.
  Fry observed, "You can laugh a lot more times a day
  than you can do push-ups."

• Sound the letters M and N, **mmmm ... nnnnn ...** ,
  as you breathe **out** long and slow. You will feel a
  resonance from the breathing muscles in the lower
  torso. These are the ones you should be using and
  need to develop.

• If you find breathing in through the nose a problem, it is
  quite all right to breathe through your mouth. The most
  important aspect is the concentration on the LONG–
  SLOW exhalation, expelling as much air from the body
  as possible, letting shoulders and body relax.

Using Controlled Pattern Breathing
in your life

As you become familiar with this technique of Controlled Pattern
Breathing you will be able to play breathing games, by altering

your pattern to, say, breathing **out** for the count of two and in for the count of two, then four **out** and one in; six **out** and one in; 12 **out** and two in, etc. You can pause for varying counts between each exhalation and inhalation, but be sure to keep your breathing working from your diaphragm.

Lying on your side in the fetal position when you go to bed is a good position in which to practice Controlled Pattern Breathing exercises, as this is the position asthmatics often assume during an attack. If you practice the breathing exercises in the same position while you are asthma-free it will become natural and comfortable for you to breathe correctly when an attack is imminent.

You may have come across similar breathing techniques already in your life: diaphragm breathing exercises are used at pre-natal classes and controlled diaphragmatic breathing is an integral part of yoga and t'ai chi. Natural therapists are usually familiar with the principles of controlled breathing, so if you are concerned about whether you are doing it right it might help you to seek some assistance from a reputable practitioner.

Breathing exercises will enable you to control and coordinate your breathing and relax your muscles, increase your air supply and strengthen your abdominal muscles. Work at it! **Breathe away your asthma**. Take every opportunity to practice Controlled Pattern Breathing so that it becomes a way of life. You will find your asthma attacks will not be as frequent as they used to be, and if you adopt this relaxation and Controlled Pattern Breathing when an attack is imminent it is less likely to become acute.

Exercising to Breathe Correctly

You now know how to breathe properly, but it still may not seem natural. This may be because your muscles just aren't ready to do the work you want them to: your body is so used to breathing from the upper chest that it tries to revert to its bad old ways as soon as you stop concentrating on it.

The following exercise regimen is not designed to get you fit (although there is a fitness exercise schedule outlined in Chapter 7) but to gradually strengthen the parts of the body you use to bring air into your lower lungs. Because your body is being re-educated after a lifetime of improper breathing habits it will probably display signs of resistance.

If you are performing the exercises correctly you might find that you are wheezing or coughing after you exhale. This may cause some initial distress. Like most new exercise, you can feel worse before you feel better! Persevere but **don't** overexert yourself or let the wheeze extend for too long. You will learn to breathe out just short of creating a wheeze. As your airways and breathing capacity improve the restricted feeling in your chest will decrease and your body will be filled with life-giving oxygen.

The breathing pattern exercises are divided into progressive steps.

1 Simple exercises to help you relax any time during the day and before you start further exercises.
2 Controlled diaphragm exercises which should be performed two or three times throughout the day when you are feeling well, and particularly before meals.

- **These exercises should only be carried out when you are feeling asthma-free** – use common sense.
- Breathe in through your nose, preferably, and **out** through the mouth making a **puhhh** sound.
- When breathing in, keep your chest muscles relaxed and the upper part of your chest still so that the breathing is performed mainly by the diaphragm.
- When breathing **out**, your whole chest should be completely relaxed, and your waist will become smaller as your stomach sinks in.
- All exercises should start and finish with breathing **out**, and be performed slowly and steadily.
- Concentrate on breathing **out**, and let breathing in be simply an automatic, reflex action. Breathing **out** should take twice as long as breathing in.
- Clear the nose often.
- Have a relaxed posture: don't hunch your shoulders.

3 More difficult exercises you can progress to when your breathing capacity has improved.

If you want to gain the most beneficial results from the exercises, each exercise should be done 6–8 times, and as often as possible throughout the day. Many of the exercises can be practiced when sitting, driving, walking, running, climbing stairs or watching television. Remember, it takes more muscular effort to be tense than it does to relax. Lessen the strain – relax.

All these exercises should only be done when you are asthma-free. Do not over-extend your breathing or exercises to the point of wheezing as **it is very important to avoid an asthma attack at any cost**, even if this means resorting to your medication or puffer.

SIMPLE RELAXATION BREATHING EXERCISES

1 Follow the relaxation exercise on page 46 but concentrate on breathing **out** long and slow and breathing in short.
2 Walk for approximately 10–15 minutes, three or four times a day if you can. While walking, practice breathing **out** for a count of two and in for a count of two, without overexerting. Extend this, where possible, to four **out** and two in; then six **out** and two in; eight **out** and two in; ten **out** and two in; and so on.

You can develop this technique by taking two steps breathing **out** and one step breathing in, then four steps **out** and one in, etc., until you reach (gradually, remember) 12 steps breathing **out** and one step breathing in.

Walking should be a relaxing and enjoyable pastime and is the best overall exercise you can do. Don't be in a hurry. Keep your breathing pattern even, stay within the limits of your airways and avoid taking deep, fast breaths high in the chest. Do not overexert yourself and possibly trigger an asthma attack.

Take your time to achieve any sustained breathing pattern. It may be two or three months before you can extend to a count **out** of ten or more. But as your fitness improves you will find that you will be able to walk for more than 15 minutes, even for several hours, without any breathing difficulties. Walk calm – walk tall.

Alice Sinclair, a 55-year-old woman, could not walk more than 200 meters without puffing, let alone climb stairs or walk up a hill. Since being introduced to Controlled Pattern Breathing she no longer has difficulty in walking or climbing stairs. In fact Alice is now running, something she thought she would never be able to do again.

CONTROLLED DIAPHRAGM EXERCISES

Rib and diaphragm exercise

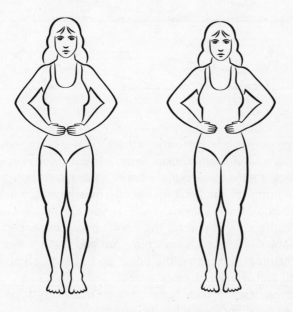

Breathing out.   Breathing in.

▶ In a sitting or standing position, with back straight, place hands on your lower ribs and push your waist in, to expel as much air as possible from the lungs. When breathing in, your hands will be forced outward by the intake of air.

▶ Push hands in as you breathe **out** and allow hands to expand as you breathe in. Don't breathe with your upper chest but use your stomach and diaphragm to do all the work. This may sound confusing and is probably the opposite to your concept of breathing but remember: breathing **out** – stomach (and diaphragm) goes in; breathing **in** – stomach (and diaphragm) out.

Diaphragm control exercise

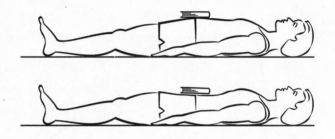

▶ Lie comfortably flat on your back on the floor, legs straight and slightly apart, arms just out from your sides. Place a light book slightly below your navel. Focus your attention on the book and gently breathe **out**, allowing the book to sink down slowly as you exhale. As you breathe in gently, push the book up as high as you can. Allow 6–10 seconds breathing **out** and 2–4 seconds breathing in, keeping the upper part of your chest as still and relaxed as possible.
▶ Repeat several times but do not be in a hurry – take your time and rest when necessary.

This exercise demonstrates rather effectively that you are using your diaphragm.

MORE DIFFICULT EXERCISES

Chest exercise

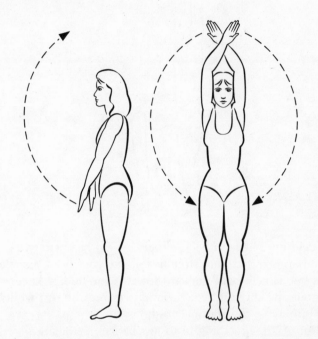

- Stand upright, hands hanging loosely and crossed in front of your body.
- Slowly raise arms in front of you to above your head, keeping your hands crossed, while breathing **out**.
  Stretch hands above the head, slowly lower your arms out to the side to a horizontal position, level with your shoulders; continue moving arms down and return to the crossed starting position, still breathing **out**. Rest.

You can vary this exercise by reversing the arm movement, or moving your arms alternately as if you were swimming backstroke. Repeat as many times as is comfortable. Don't be concerned if you hear any crackling noises in your shoulders or spine, they are just movements in the joints.

Toe touching

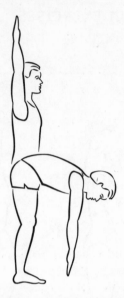

- ▶ Stand upright with back, shoulders and head straight and arms raised fully stretched above your head. Exhale as you slowly bend forward towards the floor – knees should be slightly bent. Continue to breathe **out** while returning to the starting position.
- ▶ Rest. Allow breathing in to just happen automatically.
- ▶ Repeat exercise, breathing **out** all the way to the floor and back to the starting position.

Take your time so that it takes around 5–10 seconds to complete each toe touching.

Note Watch out for vertigo (dizziness) and stop immediately if this occurs.

Sit ups

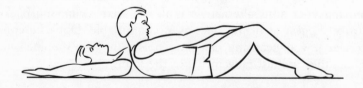

- Lie on your back on the floor with your arms and hands stretched out behind your head, knees bent, feet flat on floor.
- Raise your body slowly and start breathing **out**; bend forward until your fingers touch your knees. Breathe **out** all the way.
- Return to the original position while continuing to exhale.
- Rest, and repeat several times. Allow breathing to happen naturally.

The exercise should take 5–10 seconds to accomplish and be performed as many times as you can, up to a limit of 20 times. **Note** **The toe touching and sit up exercises can place strain on your spine so be careful if you have a sensitive back problem. If this applies to you it is wise to do some counter-balancing movements after the sit-ups to offset the extension of bending forward. You can do this by placing your hands on the lower part of your buttocks and slowly sliding your hands down your thighs as far as you can as you lean backwards, flexing your spine. Return to upright position, by moving your hands back up until you reach the starting position again breathing out continuously. Repeat a few times.**

Leg stretching

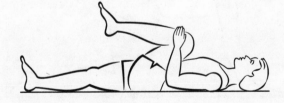

- ▶ Lie on your back, bend one leg and gently raise towards your chest.
- ▶ Clasp both hands round your knee and pull the knee as far as you can into your chest, breathing **out** for the count of 2, 4 or 6 seconds (increase the time as you become practiced at the exercise).
- ▶ Release your leg, lower to floor slowly, relax.
- ▶ Repeat with the other leg.
- ▶ Repeat whole exercise five or six times. Don't think about breathing in, just let it happen naturally.

This exercise can be extended to bending both knees and pulling them together into the chest, releasing and repeating two or three times and breathing **out** through the pulling-in movement. Practice the exercise with one knee at a time, though, before trying it with both knees.

This is also a very good back exercise and, as your flexibility increases, you might like to progress to lifting your head from the floor and bringing it towards your knees.

Squats

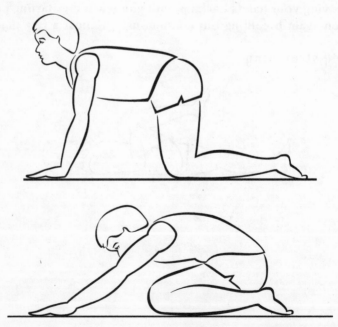

▶ Kneel on all fours and, while breathing **out**, slowly
  squat back onto your heels, keeping hands on floor,
  arms stretched out and head bent.
▶ Return to starting position, breathing in.
▶ Repeat five times.

ENJOYING DIAPHRAGM CONTROL

When you gain confidence in the breathing techniques and the
exercises above, have some fun and play diaphragm control
games. Push your diaphragm out as you breathe in and vary the
breathing pattern, always ensuring that the **out** breath is longer
than the in. See how high you can raise your diaphragm.

Try playing breathing games. Blow an object that will roll
easily, such as a pencil or table tennis ball, along a low table
from either a standing, kneeling or sitting position. Use long,
gentle breaths, concentrating on breathing **out** long and slowly.
Compete with a friend to see who can blow the object the far-
thest; or while sitting at opposite ends from a partner try to blow
the object past the other person and off the table as they blow
it back towards you. No leaning over the table – your head must
not go beyond the edge and, no cheating, you must keep your
hands behind your back, too.

Learn to play a musical wind instrument such as a trumpet,
saxophone, flute or harmonica – they all necessitate blowing,
concentration on breathing **out** and breath control. Choose an
instrument you enjoy listening to and can carry around easily.
The music you like and your age will probably govern your
choice. Some adults may lean towards the mellow tones of the
clarinet while others prefer the triumphant sounds of the
trumpet.

Blow up balloons or blow whistles. Forcefully blowing a
whistle acts like a vacuum cleaner to rid your lungs of toxic dirt
and grime. Buy a cheap whistle (remove the pea if it is too noisy
for you and your neighbors) and whistle while you work!

Christie Loughridge, a young asthma patient, demonstrated
at a recent seminar the following rather clever improvisation.

▶ Stand normally and place a large towel or belt around
  your waist, crossed over in the front of your body.

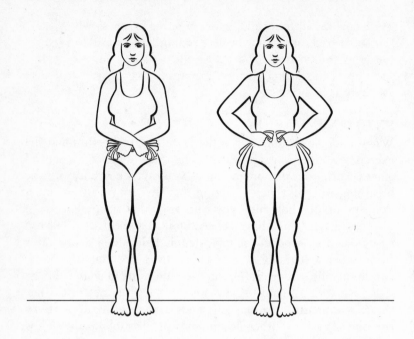

Hold the right-hand side of the towel or belt in your left hand and the left side of the towel or belt in your right hand. Simply pull on each end of the towel or belt. This pulls your stomach in and forces air out. Hold in this position for a count of 2–10, depending on your progress, then allow the towel or belt to loosen as you breathe in. Repeat as often as is comfortable. Let breathing in happen naturally.

Controlled Pattern Breathing for Children

As the parent of an asthmatic child you will need to understand just what Controlled Pattern Breathing is and its expected results. So that you are completely familiar with the concept read the detailed instructions on Learning to Relax and Controlled Pattern Breathing for adults before you start trying to teach your child.

As you will see, the instructions are far too comprehensive and complicated for children, but following is a modified version, adapted to help you and your child.

Relaxing Children

As all parents know, it is not easy to get a child to relax, but as with adults it is best if you can do so before working on their breathing. Here are some ideas that may help. Remember also the tip about teaching your child to float in a swimming pool as this helps them understand what it is you want when you ask them to relax.

THE ELEPHANT WALK

Imitating the slow, swaying, relaxed movement of an elephant moving his trunk from side to side can help very young children understand relaxation. Have the child pretend to be an elephant. Bending their knees, drooping their head forward, relaxing their shoulders, with their arms hanging loosely almost touching the floor, have them visualize and imitate an elephant slowly walking, swaying from side to side. Actually, it's fun – try it.

MONKEY FUN

The monkey is another agile animal which displays freedom of movement and an easy, relaxed attitude. Children just love to pretend they are monkeys so it's not difficult to get their co-operation to play this game. Sometimes simply crawling on the floor can loosen and relax limbs and free body movement.

Encouraging Controlled Pattern Breathing

With children below the age of five it is nigh on impossible to have them participate in Controlled Pattern Breathing exercises: they are usually too busy playing and exploring their world.

As the attention span of preschoolers is limited, you will have to turn the Breathing Pattern into a game by talking to them about "blowing up" their tummy and making it BIG, BIG, BIG. Then show them how to slowly blow **out** as much air as they can, making the short **puhhh puhhh, puhhh** sounds through their mouth. Tell them to watch how their tummy goes in and see how little they can make it. Have them try to make their tummy really BIG and really SMALL. Encourage them: aren't they clever!

Having an asthmatic child do this just once or twice every day would be quite an achievement, but if you could also have them briefly hold their breath in by asking them to see how long they can make their tummy stay BIG, it would be even better. If it is fun for them to do you are more likely to maintain their cooperation. Join in – show them how big and how small you can make your tummy and develop your own diaphragmatic breathing at the same time!

There are some wonderful games to play that will encourage children to breathe **out** long and slow. They all love blowing bubbles in the bath or with bubble pipes. Blowing a table tennis ball or pencil across a table is a fun game and can be varied by blowing through a straw. Even blowing crumbs off the table will make them happy – if you don't mind sweeping up the mess.

Children love to make a noise and although parents will have to tolerate the cacophony of sound, blowing a mouth organ, whistle or toy trumpet gives them the freedom to enjoy a pleasurable activity and exercise their airways at the same time.

Although blowing **out** in bursts with lips pursed – **puhhhh** – should be the aim of most games, little children enjoy imitating many sounds. Keep them amused pretending to be a train. They can push air out using a pattern of as many **ch, ch, ch, ch** sounds as they can, with the breaths in time with the wheels of the train along the track.

Letting children practice blowing out candles – so they can show everyone how well they can do it when their birthday arrives – is a great way to encourage them to breathe **out** long and slow. As a child develops and breathing capacity improves, this game can be expanded by increasing the distance between the child and the candle. Later they should learn to control their breath so the flame moves gently but does not go out. Sustaining this sort of breathing control, for even a minute or so a day, will improve their respiratory development.

Use your initiative and devise other suitable games and

activities, but remember the emphasis must be on breathing **out** to encourage overall relaxation and to help loosen the child's upper chest area. Be careful not to overdo these games because extended expiration can cause the child to develop a wheeze. Breathing **out**, or the **puhhh**, **puhhh** puffing, should stop just short of a wheeze. If a wheeze occurs, stop the game as it could perhaps trigger an attack. Often a cough will help to clear a wheeze and the game can continue.

Take a few minutes each day to play diaphragm breathing games with your child. Ensure it is stress-free. You can continue for as long as the child's attention span will happily permit. The important fact is that you know your child is doing controlled, diaphragmatic breathing to help expand his or her airways, even if the child doesn't.

Older children will also enjoy playing these games but they should be encouraged to have a more structured Controlled Pattern Breathing program. Asthmatic children should learn as early as possible how to cope with and manage their condition. Without turning it into a regimented discipline, they should do some diaphragmatic breathing practice each day, even for just a few minutes. Some children may be receptive to doing regular breathing exercises before or after they get out of bed in the morning, while others may prefer to do them before going to sleep. Be flexible, vary their Controlled Pattern Breathing time to suit their daily lives and to make it a pleasurable routine for you and your child.

Activities for Asthmatic Children

The best activity for your asthmatic child is learning to swim or float. Floating encourages relaxation. It is impossible to float when tense or uptight: floating can only take place when one is calm and relaxed. Learning to float helps a child experience the weightlessness of their body and overcome any fear they might have of putting their face under water. Floating is simply a matter of lying on the back with body straight and relaxed and head held well back – wriggling the toes helps keep the body afloat. A flotation board is reassuring for children to start with and will boost their confidence in the water. Having learned to float effortlessly, a child will be more receptive to learning to swim.

Follow the swimming guidelines outlined in Chapter 7 to ensure your child is competent in the water and that they follow the breathing pattern they are taught. Asthmatic children have a tendency to swim with their heads out of the water. This should most definitely be discouraged and they must concentrate on breathing **out** beneath the water.

Learning to play a musical wind instrument will teach an asthmatic child to breathe **out** LONG. There are so many choices – trumpet, clarinet, oboe, recorder or flute. The age of the child will probably govern their choice of instrument and type of music. Singing is also wonderful experience for diaphragmatic control and, who knows, you may also discover you have a child with lots of musical talent!

Sports and physical activities such as bike riding, tennis, basketball and volleyball, hockey, gymnastics, dancing, soccer, softball and baseball will not only give your asthmatic child the pleasure of participating but also develop confidence in his ability to cope with his condition, and techniques to maintain a balanced and healthy body.

Generally, in Ron's practice he has found that children's asthmatic conditions improve noticeably when they take up any of these activities and learn to use their diaphragm to improve their breathing. Encourage your child to participate in at least one of these, but without undue pressure from anyone, for unless your child is completely happy and enjoys the activity, his or her enthusiasm will wane and the activity will be of little benefit. It may be necessary, of course, to try a few pursuits before finding the right one. Also, as your child grows, interests change and horizons expand to try new and exciting exploits.

Andrew, a young boy now aged 14, had suffered from asthma since he was three years old. He was always wheezing and any sporting or physical activity aggravated his asthma. His parents decided it was in his best interests not to do any physical activities at all. Andrew had natural athletic ability and desperately wanted to play sports – of any kind. He constantly pestered his parents until, through a friend, they were recommended to Ron's clinic. After six months on the Controlled Pattern Breathing program Andrew was able to enjoy ball games and participate in sporting activities, especially bike riding. He is now highly competitive and just loves playing football, volleyball and tennis. Andrew knows he must take time to warm up slowly and has learned to relax by using self-hypnosis (see Chapter 13). He starts his athletic activities slowly.

Andrew concentrates on the breathing techniques and you can actually hear the **puhhh**, **puhhh**, **puhhh** when he is breathing **out**. He has learned to ignore comments from his friends such as "What's this **puhh**, **puhh**, **puhh** business?" He now realizes that being free from asthma is more important to him than the joking of his friends. Andrew now enjoys every minute of his happy, healthy, sports-filled life.

Controlled Pattern Breathing exercises for children

- Follow the suggestions for adults on page 61: get children to blow pencils or table tennis balls across a table, either alone or competing against one another.

Over the table game for diaphragm control.

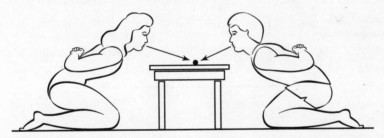

- Blowing or puffing through a straw is a great way to have fun while practicing breathing exercises. Blow or puff with a long breath **out** – **puhhh** sound – or shorter **puhhh**, **puhhh**, **puhhh**, **puhhh**, for 4–8 seconds. Breathe in short for 1–2 seconds. Breathe **out** for 4–8 seconds. Breathe in short for 1–2 seconds. Repeat as often as the child feels like it.
- Skipping, particularly with backward arm movements, strengthens and relaxes upper chest muscles and

shoulders (scapular area, pectoral, deltoids and trapezius muscles) and is an easy way for children to exercise and practice Controlled Pattern Breathing.

● Add a bit of variety to breathing exercises by having the child kneel on a padded-back chair, bending from the waist and hanging his head and upper body down over the back of the chair. It is a great way to promote air exhalation but, of course, be careful not to let the chair and child topple over!

Bending over chair to improve exhalation.

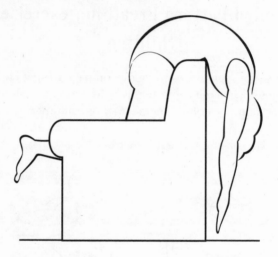

Breathing to Help Relieve
Asthma During an Attack

No doubt you will have realized by now that the breathing pattern we have been describing is directly opposite to the breathing pattern you experience during an asthma attack.

During an attack someone with asthma usually breathes heavily and quickly from the upper part of the chest. This habit tends to continue even when the attack has subsided. There is a tenseness in the upper part of the body, and the asthmatic generally finds it difficult to relax. So the first goal is to learn to **relax** during an attack. The breathing exercises below are designed to achieve this. Trying to prevent the unnatural breathing pattern of an attack is the next objective.

As an attack continues, breathing usually becomes shorter and shorter, the chest rises higher and higher with less and less air being inhaled each time, the attack becomes extreme and more and more difficult to cope with. When an asthmatic takes medication, provided it is effective, the chest starts to relax, breathing becomes easier, the breaths out become longer and slower and the diaphragm comes into play once more in the breathing process.

The purpose of Controlled Pattern Breathing, which should be practiced when asthma-free, is to help you to breathe the **opposite way** to how you breathe during an attack, so that **you** can take control of your breathing pattern by using the diaphragm and not just relying on the upper chest. The result is that instead of a distressing effort to gasp for air, with the intake becoming less and less, you can turn this breathing pattern around by concentrating on breathing **out** a little further each time and allow breathing in just to happen.

The reason for the emphasis on breathing **out** is that during an attack there is a tendency to exaggerate breathing in, to compensate for the shortness of breath. However, you should be trying to empty the chest and raise and lower the diaphragm by voluntary contraction of the abdomen and lower chest, thereby reversing the unnatural breathing of the attack. Asthmatics who breathe in heavily are generally capable of expanding the upper chest to its fullest, but by concentrating on breathing **out** and using the abdominal muscles, they will breathe more from the diaphragm, in a similar way to a singer, athlete or a swimmer.

When performing Controlled Pattern Breathing during an attack, **do not** try to change the breathing rate too quickly. It may take five, ten, 15 or even 20 minutes before the changed method of breathing is effective.

Changing the way you breathe is not easy during an attack. **This is why it is important to practice the correct breathing pattern while feeling well and asthma-free.**

Any wheeze you might develop should not be extended for more than one or two seconds. You will find that the wheeze becomes less as the expirations gradually become longer. A good cough often brings up some mucus and more than likely will help lessen the wheeze. When breathing normally, the diaphragm should be moving up and down freely.

You will have noticed if your medication is effective during an asthma attack, that your pattern of breathing changes. Remembering this, you can understand just what is expected from these breathing techniques. The breathing pattern you are being encouraged to develop is basically what occurs when a relieving medication is taken.

Remember, this breathing pattern is a method of relief, not a cure.

Just below you will find a further section on breathing exercises. These are for use in an asthma attack. However, you should continue to practice your Controlled Pattern Breathing exercises daily on a permanent basis, even if you have been free from asthma for months or years.

Relieving Asthma Attack Exercises

1   When you detect any sign that your asthma is worsening try to **relax**. Lie on your side, preferably in a comfortable bed, with your head bent forward and your knees pulled up as near as possible to your chest. Gently contract the abdomen while breathing **out**. Breathe **out** and in, maintaining a constant and even breathing pattern. Place one hand below your navel and gently push your hand in as you breathe **out**. As your breathing becomes easier, gradually extend the breathing **out**. Depending on the level of your asthma, it could take 20 minutes or more before you can change your breathing pattern.

This is probably the most effective way of relieving asthma. Do not worry too much about your poor postural position as this will correct itself once you fall asleep. And you probably will, as the effort involved in pushing air **out** will make you tired, encouraging relaxation and sleep.

Fetal position.

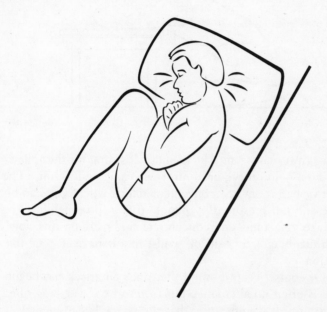

2 Especially for relief during an attack.
Kneel on the floor and rest your arms and head on a very low table or chair. Concentrate on breathing **out** slowly while gently sinking your stomach in. Then let your stomach relax while air enters the lower lungs and diaphragm without effort. In an attack your breathing rate may need to be quicker than is optimal, with the **out** and in breaths of equal duration. Gradually let your breathing become slower and more natural. Relax your shoulders and chest – put the upper part of your chest "to sleep." Take the exercise very slowly; do not over-exert or create too great a wheeze. Breathe **out** just short of wheezing.

Relieving asthma position.

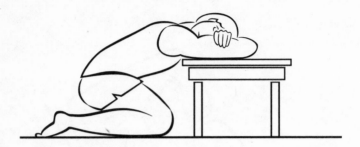

Although it may seem a little unusual, sitting on the toilet can often help relieve or control wheezing and asthma. The toilet or bathroom is a convenient refuge where you can be alone and not pressured by people trying to be helpful. You can take your time, and concentrate on breathing **out** slowly using diaphragmatic control, whilst in a bent over, fetal like position.

Of course, keep in mind that once an attack has begun, there is often no alternative but to resort to your prescribed medication. It is imperative that the attack be stopped at all costs – whether or not a drug is used. Medication generally has the ability to relax the bronchial tubes, although this, in effect, is what Controlled Pattern Breathing intends to achieve naturally. If you cannot control your attack with the Controlled Pattern Breathing you **must take your medication**.

Avoiding Attacks

Here are some suggestions that may help you avoid attacks.

- Learn to relax whether sitting or standing; at intervals relax your shoulders and let your head drop gently towards your chest.
- Keep your nasal passages clear.
- Sleep with a low, nonallergenic pillow and mattress if possible.
- Begin an exercise regimen or sports training, and slowly work your body up to higher physical fitness.
- Start and finish all exercises breathing **out**.
- Shower or bathe daily (we breathe through our skin, too).
- Add Epsom salts or essential oils to the bath water to help your muscles relax after exercise.

Buteyko Method

This is one of a number of theories advocating breathing techniques to assist asthma. Devised by Professor Buteyko of Siberia, this program consists of specific relaxation techniques and shallow breathing to correct breathlessness and wheezing. The breathing pattern is adjusted using short breaths so the asthmatic can tolerate higher than usual carbon dioxide levels in the lungs. The program aims for a short in-and-out breathing pattern which develops diaphragmatic breathing.

The Buteyko Method concentrates on not breathing through the mouth at all. It involves pinching the nose, holding the breath for as long as possible, then releasing the nose slowly so that air is expelled very slowly through it. One can draw the conclusion that it acts in a similar way to breathing in and out of a paper bag for hyperventilation. The technique requires relaxation and it is necessary to attend the program for six sessions to grasp the Buteyko concept fully.

Orthodox medicine tends to be sceptical of "miracle cures" such as the Butekyo Method, but studies of it have been funded.

One such study by an asthma foundation found that there was

> significant reduction in symptoms and the use of reliever medication in
> the Buteyko group compared with the control group after 12 weeks of
> treatment. There was also some improvement in the quality of life, with
> some participants symptom-free at the end of the study. All subjects con-
> tinued using preventer medication, although some in the Buteyko group
> were able to reduce dosage. There was no evidence of improved lung
> function in either group, and no change in carbon dioxide levels. Although
> this study shows benefits for 90 per cent of the Buteyko group, the reasons
> are as yet unknown and warrant further research. If people do try Buteyko,
> and other treatments, we still recommend continuing with the medications
> prescribed by their doctor. A complementary approach with support of
> your doctor and your asthma action plan is still the best and safest option.

If reactions from participants are any indication, the Butekyo
Method is proving very beneficial for some severe asthmatics. It
would seem that most people who have attended a course are
pleased with the improvement in their asthma and have lessened
their reliance on medication. However, the Butekyo program is
costly, which may not make it an available option for some.

Sarah is a six-year-old girl who suffers from chronic asthma.
Her mother, Michelle, had tried everything in the way of orthodox treatment for her but Sarah still needed to go to the hospital
on a weekly basis for treatment for her asthma. After attending
the Buteyko program, Sarah showed at least a 70 per cent
improvement. Her mother was so pleased with the result that
she is now committed to promoting the method.

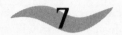

PHYSICAL EXERCISE

At the 1984 Olympic Games in Los Angeles, 20 per cent of the athletes competing had asthma, and this percentage is reflected in many sports. Swimming may even have a higher number of asthmatics than this, as swimming is recommended for children with asthma. Among the many prominent asthmatics who have reached the top in their particular sport are Jackie Joyner-Kersey, the American track star, Adrian Moorhouse, the world-record holding British breaststroke swimmer, and cricket stars Allan Border from Australia and Ian Botham from England.

Generally sportsmen and women believe that the training they undergo and the exercise they take improves their asthma. It is also true that in training they learn to breathe as efficiently as possible to maximize their sports potential — using those all-important diaphragm muscles to control their breathing patterns!

A misconception has certainly existed in the past, and may still be found today, that people with asthma cannot or should not exercise at all. The belief behind this is that even minimal exercise will trigger an attack. However, with rare exceptions, all asthmatics can and should participate in a carefully chosen, planned and monitored exercise program. We do not suggest that asthma can be "cured" by physical exercise, but it certainly can be managed and controlled while exercising, and the resultant improvement in physical fitness will improve the asthmatic's health. Everyone, asthmatic or not, should regularly take 30 minutes a day to exercise all parts of their body. If they did it would certainly result in a healthier world.

Whether or not you intend – or are able – to take up a sport, you should still try to keep yourself fit. Below we set out a daily exercise program that is not time-consuming or stressful, but if regularly performed will have a definite, positive effect on your asthma. If you are in any doubt about whether you should be attempting these exercises talk to your doctor before starting the program. Don't rush into it, either: you should build up your fitness gradually. Do not over-extend yourself while exercising. If you feel strained, tired or uncomfortable, review your program, cut out the steps that are too difficult at the moment and lessen the number of times you perform an exercise until you can build your fitness to an improved level. And, of course, don't push yourself to a point where you bring on an asthma attack.

A Daily Exercise Program

The most difficult thing about an exercise regimen or physical pursuit is "putting on your shoes," in other words – getting started!

A good level of physical fitness and a healthy mental attitude (yes, exercise **does** improve your state of mind as it makes you more alert and lifts depression) requires a regular breathing and exercise routine lasting 15–20 minutes every morning. We say the morning, as this is when you will feel the most benefit from the exercise, carrying its energizing effects with you for the rest of the day, and we have devised a program that starts from the moment you wake up.

Don't look upon the exercises we describe below as the **only** ones you should be doing, as you can modify the program to suit your particular needs. It is more important that you exercise daily and that you enjoy what you are doing. The exercises you do need not be strenuous, just simple and practical, but should involve movements of extension and flexibility.

Begin the exercises slowly, remembering to breathe **out**, using the Controlled Pattern Breathing we described in Chapter 6, during the maximum effort of the exercise. For example, when doing a push up, breathe **out** all the way through the push up. Rest – then breathe in short – and continue the exercise breathing **out** for 2, 4, 6, 8 or 10 seconds and breathing in for 2, depending on your ability and level of breath control. The same principle applies to any exercise – be it riding a bike, leg raisers, push ups, leg squats or arm swings.

Before starting your exercise remember the following rules:

- breathe **out** long and slow to start the exercise
- breathe **out** long and slow to finish the exercise
- always breathe long **out**, short in
- do the exercises slowly and carefully – do not hurry the movements
- monitor yourself so that you do not aggravate your asthma
- relax and rest after each exercise.

EXERCISES

1 On waking, concentrate on diaphragmatic controlled breathing. Place your hands flat on your stomach slightly below the navel and, as you press down with your hands, breathe **out** while being aware that the stomach goes in. Breathe in, allowing the hands to rise and the stomach to expand. Continue breathing slowly at the pattern you have built up, always aiming to breathe **out** for longer than you breathe in.
Initially just practise breathing for about a minute or so, and build up to 5–10 minutes every morning. Concentrate on breathing **out** and allowing breathing in to happen naturally.

2 Before getting out of bed, gently stretch your whole body – pretend you are a cat. Then, with both arms above your head and legs straight, stretch your left arm and right leg as far as you can. Relax; now stretch your right arm and left leg. Do this 2–3 times, relax and let your body go limp, breathing **out** long and slow.

3 Lie on your back, legs straight, and while breathing **out** gently bend one leg up towards your chest. Breathe in short. Slowly stretch leg straight, breathing **out** as you stretch. Repeat 5 times for each leg.

4 Slowly roll out of bed sideways, stand, rotate your arms backwards or forwards in wide circles – windmill fashion – for about 20–30 seconds. Breathe **out** as you bring your arms up and in as your arms swing down. Take 2–3 seconds to complete each circle.

5 March on the spot about 20 times, raising each knee as high as you can towards your chest, breathing long **out**, short in.

6 With arms horizontally stretched out in front of your body, breathe **out** as you slowly move your arms backwards as far as you can and then, breathing in, bring palms forward until they are together. Relax. Repeat 5 times.

7 Start with arms at your sides. Move them outwards and upwards in an arc to above your head, while breathing **out**. Lower your arms to your sides, breathe in and relax. Repeat 5 times.

8 Move your head gently in different directions: sideways, forwards, backwards, and rotate slowly to the left and the right. This is very relaxing and will improve the flexibility in your neck and shoulders and release any tension.

9 With hands on hips, rotate your body by turning from the hips. Bend forward towards the toes, turn your body to the right, flex backwards, then to the left and return to the starting position. Repeat 3–5 times, rotating left to right and right to left, breathing **out** long and slow and in short.

10 After performing the upright exercises, gradually move to the floor by bending your knees and crouching up and down a few times to flex your joints.

11 Kneel on all fours, then raise left leg and right arm together and push away from your body, just like a cat stretching. Alternate with right leg and left arm and repeat 3–5 times each side. No need to hurry, but

do think about breathing **out** while you are lazily
stretching.

12 Lie on your front and do push-ups, either from the
knees or if you are able to, the feet. Breathe **out**
during each push up, then relax and allow breathing in
just to happen. You may only be able to achieve a few
push ups, but do as many as you can, remembering to
breathe **out**. Stop, rest and relax before continuing.

13 Turn onto your side, do 5–10 side leg raises each side,
breathing **out** as you raise your leg and in as you
lower it.

14 Lie on your back flat on the floor with arms and legs
outstretched. Raise arms and legs off the floor
alternately – or together if you can – 1–5 times.
Breathe **out** as you raise your hands and feet and in as
you lower them to the floor.

15 While on your back do sit ups – breathe **out** as you
perform each sit up and in when completed. If you
can't manage sit ups simply rock back and forth with
both knees tucked up into your chest. This is also a
great back exercise.

16 Rest and relax with Controlled Pattern Breathing.

IMMUNE SYSTEM ACTIVATOR

The importance of a having a healthy immune system to neu-
tralize or destroy any microorganisms that attack the body has
been discussed already in this book. There is an exercise you can
do to improve your immune system.

In the middle of the upper chest, where the top ribs join
the breastbone (sternum) is a nut-shaped organ called the thymus
gland. The thymus is a vital part of the extensive lymphatic
system, which makes up a large part of the immune system.
Using a Tarzan-like action, gently tap or pat this area for 10–15
seconds, 2–3 taps per second, each day after your exercise program, to stimulate the gland. You will also help loosen phlegm
by doing this – useful for people with asthma, who tend to have
a buildup of mucus in their respiratory systems.

Exercise-induced Asthma

Exercise-triggered asthma occurs when cold or dry air enters the airways. Continuous, strenuous activity causes rapid breathing through the mouth and the air that reaches the air passages is not warmed and humidified by the nose and upper airways as it is with normal breathing through the nose. For instance, while jogging, air is inhaled rapidly through the mouth, the airways dry out and the result is often asthma symptoms. Any exercising outdoors during cold weather or in a cold, dry environment is likely to cause asthma in sensitive individuals so activities such as ice skating and skiing should be avoided by them.

Even if you are prone to exercise-induced asthma, choosing the right type of exercise and using pre-exercise breathing techniques will help you prevent triggering an attack. Just because a particular physical activity or exercise aggravates your asthma it does not necessarily mean you should avoid further participation. Instead, the exercise may need to be modified and your program adapted to the limits of your condition.

Exercise-triggered symptoms usually subside within several minutes, but can sometimes still be evident up to one hour after exercise. Be cautious during this time – and take medication if necessary to prevent your condition deteriorating.

Most asthmatics' degree of well-being varies from day to day or season to season, so select a varied exercise program to accommodate the highs and lows of your condition. If your breathing tubes have narrowed or become blocked it will be difficult for you to blow out hard and strenuous exercise will be uncomfortable. A light workout, such as walking, will still do you the world of good. Use a peak flow meter on a daily basis so that you can adjust your exercise program as necessary.

There appears to be a general pattern that exercise-induced asthma develops about 5–10 minutes into the exercising, which is sometimes known as "second-wind stage;" it may also appear 5–10 minutes after the exercise has stopped. It has been found that if athletes take care to do a thorough warm-up routine before they begin the serious exercise the chances of developing asthma are greatly reduced. Likewise, warm down slowly from strenuous activity.

If you do find that you are wheezing and are short of breath you must take care not to trigger an attack, although remember that panting may be the result of the normal exercise and is not necessarily asthma. Correct breathing may avert the asthma but if asthma does develop, take your prescribed medication, remembering that attacks must be avoided.

Second Wind – the Critical Stage

People often find that the first few minutes of physical effort are a danger time. After starting exercise everyone, asthmatic or not, reaches a point of feeling breathless – the second-wind stage. However, asthmatics can quickly deteriorate from normal panting to severe wheezing, shortness of breath and an attack.

It is possible to force yourself through this danger point and get your second wind with Controlled Pattern Breathing. The key is maintaining steady, consistent diaphragmatic breathing right from the beginning of the activity, to decrease the suddenness of the second-wind stage. No matter how much you feel like taking a deep breath you must try not to, so that you can "push through" past the second-wind stage and bypass an attack.

You need not stop your exercise, but should adjust your pattern of breathing to accommodate the severity of the second-wind stage. Nor should you extend your breath to the point of wheezing. With lips loose, breathe **out puhhh**, to just short of a wheeze. Breathing **out** for 2 seconds and in for 2 seconds, or **out** for 4 seconds and in for 2 seconds, will probably take you to just short of a wheeze and is usually all the effort you need to get you through to your second wind. It may be necessary to maintain this breathing pattern for 5 minutes, but sometimes even up to an hour, before you feel comfortable.

Take it easy to start with, but keep your diaphragmatic breathing pattern even. Try not to alter this breathing routine, no matter how exhausting it might seem at the beginning. Having taken yourself through the second-wind stage, breathing will become more natural and easier.

Obviously you should have learned Controlled Pattern Breathing and be practicing it regularly before you try to use it during exercise, when an asthma attack may be triggered. It does require discipline in the early stages to control the urge to over-breathe and gulp air into the chest. Of course, if you cannot adjust your breathing pattern while exercising and you feel you might trigger an asthma attack, stop what you are doing imme-diately. If possible, lie in the fetal position and concentrate on performing Controlled Pattern Breathing. However, an asthma attack must be avoided, so **take your medication** if this is necessary.

Julian, a twelve-year-old boy, could not walk for more than 200 meters without puffing and panting, much less do anything more strenuous. Just walking upstairs or climbing a hill was daunting for him. Julian worked hard at learning Controlled Pattern Breathing and how to push through the second-wind barrier to overcome breathlessness. The result is that he can now walk many kilometers and only becomes physically exhausted as a result of muscle tiredness.

Sports

It is imperative that you start any sporting or physical activity slowly, building gradually to peak performance. Always warm up slowly and gradually. Your warm-up routine should take **twice as long** as nonasthmatics'. While warming up concentrate on breathing using the Controlled Pattern Breathing in Chapter 6.

Once you have warmed up thoroughly you can increase the pace of the exercise as long as your breathing pattern is able to keep up. Again, you should concentrate on breathing **out** as much as possible. While exercising only **you** will know just how far you can go without aggravating your condition. Do not allow your breathing to become distressed.

A warm up should involve gradually stretching and loos-ening all the muscles you will be using. Whatever the sport, try to include some exercises for arms and shoulders. Ideal move-ments are the actions used in freestyle and backstroke swimming – "windmill" arm rotations. These loosen and strengthen the upper dorsal region of the body, which in turn exercises the trapezius and pectoral muscles. The result will be a strengthening and development of the chest, with resultant better alignment of the vertebrae in the spine and alleviation of any nerve impingement.

No specific sports program is recommended in this book, as the best sport for anyone will depend on the individual. However, before taking up a new sport discuss it with your doctor, who may wish to assess your physical capabilities first.

Which Sport?

Acquiring skills of sharp coordination, agility, quick thinking and reflex reactions can be of enormous benefit to someone with asthma. The stamina that comes with physical fitness is also an asset to anyone. The training done by a boxer, gymnast or ballet dancer develops these, as well as flexibility, strength and concentration.

Boxing may seem an odd choice of activity for an asthmatic. However, consider the boxer's loud expulsion of air when throwing a punch. This expulsion of air is made during an extreme effort, similar to that of a tennis player serving a ball (Monica Seles is a memorable example of this), or a soccer player kicking the ball, an athlete leaving the blocks or a squash player making a shot. You will hear competitors in many sports make this often loud and obvious expulsion of air. It helps them relax immediately after the point of maximum impact.

The quick expulsion of air may not be exactly the same as the slower expulsion in the Controlled Breathing Pattern, but we believe that someone with asthma should choose a sport that involves breathing **out** at the time of maximum impact, or when intense effort is involved. However, sports that require longer and slower breathing **out** are even better.

Football, basketball, cricket, gymnastics, netball, volleyball and ballet are suitable for asthmatics as they require short, quick bursts of effort. In contrast long distance running, where sustained effort is needed over a considerable period, is an example of a sport that stresses asthmatics and aggravates their condition. Likewise, scuba diving, skydiving and bungee jumping are not sports we would recommend to someone with asthma.

No matter what sport is the final choice – be it table tennis, badminton, softball, horse riding or whatever — they all need agility, concentration, flexibility and strength. Regular exercise will start you on the stairway to better health, and will help your body reach its full potential and keep it there. Exercise should be dynamic, varied, accessible and without adverse side effects, and don't forget the all-important factor of choosing one you really enjoy. If you disregard this you won't keep the sport up.

Whatever the activity, always keep your limitations in mind and conscientiously follow the breathing and relaxation techniques described in Chapter 6.

Swimming

Although we do not recommend one sport above another in this book, there is no doubt that swimming is an excellent activity for people with asthma. It has been called the complete sport for asthmatics and its benefits have resulted in it being used worldwide as a treatment for asthma.

Why is it so good? Swimming's many arm movements promote upper chest development and flexibility, and therefore better breathing. The controlled breathing pattern is just what an asthmatic needs for unstressful respiratory exercise. Swimming is also environmentally suitable for someone with asthma as the air is taken in just above the water and so it is already warmed and humidified and unlikely to trigger an attack.

Further, while swimming the body weight is partially supported by the water. This means that strain and pressure on muscles and joints is lessened, which in turn promotes freedom of movement in the water. The result is that swimming involves less physical demands on the body than sports such as running or cycling. The same reason means that aqua-aerobics and hydrotherapy are also good exercise for people whose bodies, or asthma, are not able to take the strain of higher pressure sports.

Some years ago, in conjunction with the Victorian Asthma Foundation in Australia, Ron introduced a trial swimming program for asthmatics. Many of the people who participated showed such a remarkable improvement that similar programs were introduced by asthma organizations worldwide. Today, asthmatics everywhere are encouraged to take up swimming.

A successful swimming regimen may take a little time to

establish. A beginner must learn to swim, and is often apprehensive at the start. However, following the initial training, when the swimmer has gained confidence and learned to relax, the results are usually impressive.

The best environment for teaching an asthmatic to swim is a heated pool. Having a trained instructor is the optimum way to learn and he or she should be aware of the asthmatic condition. As many beginners are unfamiliar with water and are anxious, gaining confidence is an important part of learning to swim enjoyably. A relaxed approach by the instructor reassures the pupil and avoids the possibility of an anxiety-induced attack, which would only defeat the purpose of the exercise.

Once an asthmatic has learned to swim competently, he or she will also have learned the pattern of breathing **out** long underwater and taking a short breath at the surface between strokes. You will immediately recognize the similarities between this breathing and the Controlled Pattern Breathing which is the key to managing asthma.

It does not matter whether an asthmatic swims freestyle, breaststroke or backstroke, swimming should be carried out on a regular basis with a planned program, making sure you do not try too much too soon. Even though backstroke does not involve breathing **out** under the water, the breathing pattern and the arm movements are still valuable for upper chest and respiratory development.

Learning to float, especially on the back, is also useful because floating can only be achieved when the body is completely relaxed and is a sign that the student has overcome any anxiety he or she might have had to start with in the water.

Swimming isn't without its dangers, of course, as any excessive exercise or physical demands may trigger asthma. However, proper monitoring and planning should prevent overexertion. And, like any sport, a regular training schedule will result in the gradual development of strength and stamina.

Once regular training has been established, asthmatics often become so motivated and enthusiastic they take up swimming competitively. Rebecca Brown is one of them. As a child she took up swimming to help her asthma and has gone on to become a champion. Rebecca is currently the world record holder for the 200 meter breaststroke. She is dedicated to being the best, and this involves strong discipline. With ten training sessions a week she only has half a day a week to rest and relax. Her diet is also watched closely – no sweets, chocolate or soft drinks. Although Rebecca is a chronic asthmatic she deliberately plays down her condition and resorts to medication only when necessary. Coach Michael Piper says, "Asthma is the reason for her introduction to swimming at the age of four and it has never interfered with her training. She is addicted to success."

Another world record holder, Samantha Riley, who holds the shortcourse 100 and 200 meter breaststroke records, is also an asthmatic.

Young twin patients of Ron's, Andre and Paul, had both suffered from asthma since early childhood. This had severely inhibited their playing sports. They had to use their puffers daily and always needed them before any physical activity. For two years they followed a regulated swimming program and complementary Controlled Pattern Breathing regime, and their asthma improved remarkably. Their reliance on inhalers has been reduced so much that they now only carry them for psychological support.

8

DIET

Eating Well Means Good Health

Microscopic, yet potentially lethal, organisms invade us throughout our lives. Harmful bacteria and viruses can be found in or on almost everything we eat, drink, breathe or touch. Our immune system, which consists of special cells within the body, recognizes and fights these marauding invaders. Without the immune system our bodies would not cope with such constant attacks and people would die from simple ailments like the common cold. A healthy immune system is our greatest ally and good nutrition our best ammunition.

How does a healthy immune system improve asthma? In two ways. First, many people find their asthma is triggered, or worsened, by respiratory illnesses – coughs and colds. If their immune systems prevent viruses and bacteria taking hold in the body, the chances are that their asthma will improve. Secondly, the immune system plays a part in the inflammatory reaction in asthma (see page 13) and a healthy immune system may not be so ready to overreact to asthma triggers.

Nutrients and vitamins stimulate the body's immune system while deficiencies adversely affect the body in various ways. It is well known that a Vitamin C deficiency results in the body being more susceptible to respiratory illnesses such as colds. Other nutrients and trace elements are important: Vitamin E enhances the immune system, while a lack of Vitamin B6 can lower the white blood cells and reduce antibody production.

But are we feeding our immune systems properly? Sadly, the answer seems to be "No." A newspaper report in June 1994 gave the result of a survey into eating habits: it found that people were eating a wider variety of foods than they did ten years ago, but the nutritional content had not improved. The consequence of poor nutrition in the developed world is a diet-related sickness bill of billions of dollars annually.

Considering the huge and ever-increasing consumption of carbonated drinks, alcohol, canned and frozen foods in general, fried snack foods, potato chips, french fries, ice cream, hot dogs, hamburgers, chocolate and candies, is it any wonder that the health and well-being of Western societies is being affected? Add to this the increasing use of refined white flour rather than whole-grain, salt, sugar, tea and coffee, and the picture gets gloomier. Food is being heavily refined, and preservatives and artificial colorings added. Nutrients are lost from the refined end products. On top of the poor quality of the foods we *do* eat, we have been consuming fewer fruits, vegetables and herbs, which are generally high in vitamins, minerals and trace elements.

There is evidence to suggest that dietary habits are moving from bad to worse. A recent survey of secondary school children in Victoria, Australia, found that in some schools one in ten students did not eat any fruit *at all* during the month-long study. Although this was a relatively small study, it identified a problem and leads to great concern about the unbalanced food intake of growing adolescents.

Typically the children were eating fast foods and sweet bakery items during the day, while drinking sugared, colored and carbonated drinks. That such a situation can exist where one child in ten does not eat any fruit at all is a blight on our society. An abundance of fruit, such as apples, oranges, grapes and bananas, is available throughout the year at minimal cost. It would appear that our society is being conditioned to avoid fruit, and that other, less nutritious substances are being promoted in its place. It is imperative that people with asthma eat fruit, preferably three or four pieces per day, because fruit is rich in vitamins and minerals.

A Diet for Asthmatics

Hippocrates, the Greek father of medicine from the fourth century BC, summed up lifestyle and good health in a clear and forthright manner with his advice: **"Let your food be your medicine."**

To improve your general health look closely at the food you eat. If possible, eat organically grown fruit and vegetables and avoid foods with artificial additives and preservatives. The fat content and density of red meat place a strain on the digestive system, as it is difficult for the body's enzymes to break it down, but red meat is a great source of iron. For good health, though, limit the overall amount in your diet, eat small portions, chew well and always remove the fat. White meat such as fish and chicken is more digestible, but do get rid of the chicken skin first − it contains too much fat.

Do yourself a favor and throw out the frying pan. Grilling will reduce the fat content in your diet. Likewise, forget the takeouts, fast foods and overprocessed convenience foods. All they do is raise your cholesterol level and put more fat into your body. Cholesterol-free vegetable oils and margarines are readily available and are palatable alternatives for cooking.

On the other hand, essential fatty acids (EFAs) are vital components of the walls of every cell in our body. They also play parts in the biochemical processes which sustain our health and our life. An essential fatty acid deficiency can cause an imbalance of prostaglandins, substances that regulate immune cell activity and thus control inflammation and allergic reactions, both of which play a part in asthma. Disorders such as depressed immunity, eczema, poor healing of wounds, cardiovascular abnormalities and PMS have all been associated with EFA deficiencies.

Cold-pressed sunflower, safflower, linseed and soya oils, salmon, herring and mackerel or fish oil supplements and evening primrose oil are good dietary sources of EFAs. We recommend cold-pressed oils only, as oils not labeled as refined in this way will have been extracted from their source using chemicals and are not as healthy for you. Add a selection of haricot, kidney or soy beans to your diet, and nuts such as walnuts, almonds and brazil nuts (peanuts and cashews are not as useful), for a varied combination of EFAs in your diet.

EFA supplies in the body are depleted by eating processed foods, cigarette smoke, alcohol and pollution. You should be aware that margarine from polyunsaturated oils that have been hydrogenated to solidify them does not contain EFAs.

You might like to consider the benefits of a vegetarian diet. However, a vegetarian lifestyle requires a great deal of thought, planning and dedication to ensure the food intake is well balanced. For instance, if you eliminate meat from your diet you must make sure you include alternative iron-rich foods or supplements. Making such a radical change to eating habits requires strong discipline. Ask yourself: "Can I do it, how will it affect my system, and can I afford not to do it?" A consultation with your medical practitioner is advisable before coming to any decision.

Even if you don't become a vegetarian you should ensure your intake of grains, fruit and vegetables is high. One result will be improvement in your bowel movement pattern. We believe that daily bowel usage is essential for asthmatics. You may ask: "Why is improved bowel function so important to an asthmatic?" It is well recognized by naturopaths, nutritionists and dietitians that when the body eliminates excessive toxins, the liver and other organs function more efficiently. Indirectly this improves the body's metabolism and so builds up the immune system. This is a basic principle of good health. Just remember the maxim "We are tomorrow what we eat today." If you eat a diet that is high in grains, fruit and vegetables – and consequently high in roughage – better health will be the result and indirectly the likelihood of asthma will be reduced.

Roughage and fiber are naturally present in high quantities in bran, whole-grain bread, wheat germ, raisins, dates, sultanas, prunes, garlic and especially in the skin of apples and grapes. An ideal breakfast is a combination of wheat germ, bran and muesli with raw or stewed fruit. Canned fruit, without added sugar, is acceptable for the sake of convenience. All vegetables, particularly carrots, celery, potatoes, parsnip, cauliflower and broccoli, as well as herbs such as senna pod, licorice and cascara, will improve and regulate bowel function. Drinking plenty of water will soften the body's waste and make it easier to eliminate.

Foods to avoid are those most likely to cause constipation. The pies, pastries, fast foods and overrefined white foods of today's society should not be part of your regular diet.

Numerous herbal and homeopathic proprietary lines, such as nux vomica, lycopodium and china, are available from health food stores to improve bowel function, but do avoid using laxatives on a long-term basis. Your aim should be to achieve daily bowel function naturally, not through medications.

Dairy foods have a high protein content as well as containing essential vitamins and minerals, particularly calcium. However, research has indicated that eating dairy foods from cows tends to lead to over production of mucus in the respiratory passages of some people, which obstructs their breathing. Children with constantly blocked or running noses often significantly improve when they stop drinking cow's milk. This does not mean milk and related products should be eliminated entirely from an asthmatic child's diet, as soy, goat's or sheep's milk can be substituted and sheep's or goat's yogurt and cheese used. Tofu ice cream is a readily available alternative to the dairy product.

Even if you don't have an allergy to cow's produce that causes asthma many other problems have been linked to cow's milk intolerance or allergy, including eczema, sinusitis, catarrh, hay fever and gastrointestinal illnesses. It is wise to reduce or limit the amount of cheese, cream and other dairy products in the diet. Adults should restrict milk to a maximum of half a pint per day and rely on water or fruit juices for their daily fluid intake.

Because of its excessive carbohydrate content, lessen your reliance on refined sugar. Cut down on the sweet items and replace them with raisins, dates, prunes, sultanas, almonds and lots of fruit. Honey is an ideal substitute for sugar – have a spoonful of honey if you need to sweeten something. You can chew honeycomb instead of eating chocolate. Honey isn't just a sweetener, though, as international research suggests it can effectively inhibit the growth of bacteria. How this works is as yet unclear, but it would seem that everyone who has researched honey agrees that it has health benefits. Dr. Michael Wootton, associate professor in the department of food, science and technology at the University of New South Wales, Australia, takes honey and lemon for colds and believes the small amounts of acids and natural peroxide contained in honey may inhibit the growth of microorganisms.

The desire for sugared and sweetened foods can be overcome by using lemon. Before meals take a teaspoon of lemon juice in a glass of lukewarm water to adjust your taste buds. This will settle your craving for sweet things naturally! It will also prepare your body to digest other foods and assist the work of the stomach's enzymes.

Although refined white flour is normally used in bread, cakes, biscuits, pastries and so on, if these foods are a must for you then bake them with whole-grain flour.

Common table salt (sodium chloride) in excess can make you retain fluid. In moderate amounts, however, salt can actually thin out mucus in the respiratory tract. There are many tasty food enhancers such as garlic or vegetable salt, as well as combinations of spices and herbs to add zest to your cooking. Many herbs such as ginger and turmeric have anti-inflammatory properties as well.

Water is as crucial to our existence as air. Water makes up more than half of our body's weight. Our cells are full of water. Water supports all our body's processes. Water is the basis of blood, and therefore of the transport system of the body. Water collects the wastes and toxins from cells, dilutes them and carries them to our eliminating organs. Water carries oxygen to the cells to create energy. Impure or inadequate water supplies mean every cell in our body suffers.

Our body excretes about 2.5 liters of fluid per day (the equivalent of ten cups), through our skin as well as our kidneys. We must perpetually put back what we lose. The food we eat daily contains about two or three cups of fluid; metabolic water (the kind made in our cells as a result of chemical reactions) provides another cup; this leaves six or seven cups of fluid we need to drink every day. Pure, unadulterated water is the best way of getting this fluid, although fruit juices and milk – in limited quantities – are almost as good. Be careful, though, as many city water supplies are contaminated and contain inorganic substances such as lead, cadmium and chemical additives that impair our immune system. Invest in a water filter system – there are many inexpensive ones now available – and taste the difference. Try to drink at least half the recommended 6–7 glasses of liquid daily as pure water. Limit alcohol and caffeine consumption. Keep up the recommended level of liquid, too, especially as you grow older, when the thirst drive diminishes: your body's need for water does not.

Did you know that large quantities of vitamins are destroyed with inappropriate cooking methods? Review the way you prepare your meals – are you destroying your nourishment? There are many good books available on how best to cook food in order to retain its nutritional content and reduce vitamin loss, but in general steam vegetables in preference to boiling them, and be careful not to overcook grains or legumes.

Let your food be your medicine – not your medicine your food. We believe you should also follow the old saying: "Breakfast like a king, lunch like a prince and dine like a pauper." Use the following plan as a guide to keep you feeling vital and alive. *Bon appetit!*

SAMPLE MEAL PLAN

BREAKFAST   *Citrus fruit or fruit juice; whole-grain cereal and/or boiled, poached or scrambled egg.*

LUNCH   *Lean meat, poultry or fish; potato or brown rice; green vegetable, other vegetables; stewed or fresh fruit.*

DINNER   *Fish, cheese or egg; salad; fresh fruit.*

SNACKS   *Raw fruit, dried fruit, nuts, celery, carrot sticks, cheese.*

Remember to restrict butter, cream, fat, and all sugars, including brown and raw sugar, in your diet. Use salt in moderation. Use glucose syrup or honey if necessary.

A final point: although we would not generally recommend caffeine as a part of a healthy diet, it may have a place in an asthmatic's life! Allergist Allan Becker, M.D., assistant professor of medicine at the University of Manitoba, suggests that if an asthmatic feels an attack coming on and has no inhaler at hand, "a couple of cups of strong coffee will have a beneficial effect." The asthma drug theophylline is almost identical chemically to caffeine, and when asthmatics were given pills containing the amount of caffeine contained in two cups of coffee they "could breathe better and their asthma improved." However, he does caution that caffeine is not a substitute for medication: "We don't

---

recommend it as a treatment, but in an emergency when you don't have your medication around, two strong cups of coffee or hot cocoa, or a couple of chocolate bars, would be an effective substitute medication that would buy time until you could get to your medicine or inhaler."

Vitamins and Minerals in the Diet

As an asthmatic you need to ensure your diet contains plenty of vitamins and minerals, to build up your body's immune system. Here is a chart to give you some more information about the types of food you will find the vitamins in.

VITAMIN	FUNCTION	SOURCE
A	Maintains healthy skin in the linings of the lungs and intestines. Increases resistance to infection. Improves night vision.	Liver, eggs, dairy products; cod liver oil; spinach, yellow or orange vegetables such as carrot, pumpkin and sweet potato.
B1 (Thiamin)	Involved in energy-releasing reactions in the body.	Whole-grain cereals and bread; wheat germ; peas, sesame seeds, almonds, yeast (brewers and extract), meat extract.
B2 (Riboflavin)	Involved in energy-releasing reactions in the body.	Liver, kidney, yeast extract, dairy products.
B3 (Niacin)	Involved in energy-releasing reactions in the body.	Whole-grain cereals, liver, poultry, meat, tuna, peanuts.
B5 (Pantothenic acid)	Involved in energy-releasing reactions in the body and formation of red blood cells and neurotransmitters.	Liver, kidney, whole-grain products, peanuts, eggs, watermelon.
B6 (Pyridoxine)	Involved in energy-releasing reactions in the body and manufacture of proteins and red blood cells.	Whole-grain products, bananas, liver, avocado, lean meats.

B12 (Cobalamin)	Manufacture of DNA and RNA in nuclei of cells, and in substance covering nerves.	Eggs, liver, fish, oysters, meat.
Folate (Folic acid)	Manufacture of red and white blood cells and DNA. Important for growth.	Yeast, liver, dark green leafy vegetables, wheat germ.
C	Involved in growth and maintenance of connective tissue, blood vessels, bones and teeth; also in manufacture of hormones. Assists wound healing and is antioxidant.	Many fruits and vegetables, especially citrus, tomato, capsicum (in peppers), broccoli, strawberries, guava, potato, black currants.
D	Necessary for the body to absorb and use calcium, i.e. vital for bones and teeth to develop properly.	Liver, fatty fish, egg yolk, dairy products, margarine.
E	Antioxidant. Works with selenium to protect cells from damage. Has a role in healing of wounds.	Vegetable oils: wheat-germ, sunflower, olive and safflower oils; margarine, almonds, wholegrains.
Biotin (Vitamin H)	Manufacture of fatty acids and involved in metabolism of proteins and carbohydrates.	Yeast, chicken liver, soybeans, eggs, oysters, whole-grain bread, fish.
K	Ensures normal clotting of blood.	Green leafy vegetables (spinach, broccoli, cabbage), eggs, liver.

Following is a selection of those vitamins, minerals and other trace substances which should be part of your regular diet. We recommend that you also supplement your diet with extra vitamins and minerals that are of particular benefit to asthmatics, and we cover these in greater detail on pages 99–110.

Vitamin A and beta-carotene

Vitamin A, or retinol, is essential for keeping the mucous membranes lining the respiratory passages, lungs and digestive system healthy, and for good vision. It improves resistance to infection, and is necessary for bone and blood vessel growth. Vitamin A is also responsible for maintaining an active thymus gland (part of the immune system). Beta-carotene, sometimes referred to as pro-Vitamin A, is a related substance that the body can convert readily into Vitamin A.

Because of its importance in keeping the lining of the lungs healthy and in the immune system, Vitamin A is a vital part of the diet for asthmatics. It is also of use to bronchitis and sinusitis sufferers, for skin problems, stress-related problems, gastric ulcers and arthritis. Poor immunity, a reduced sense of taste and smell, night blindness, and dry skin and eyes, are signs of a Vitamin A deficiency. The best food sources of Vitamin A are animal and fish livers, kidneys, dark green and orange vegetables, egg yolk and milk. Beta-carotene is found in the yellow pigment of fruits and vegetables such as carrots.

Chlorophyll
Chlorophyll, the pigment that absorbs light energy and makes plants green, is a natural blood enhancer and neutralizer of toxins. Studies have revealed it reduces infections of the upper respiratory tract and sinuses and various types of chronic ulcers, while recent research showed that it can counteract the effects of pollution and radiation. It is included in some toothpastes and mouthwashes to curb bad breath.

Chlorophyll is found in all green plants, but seaweed, alfalfa, barley and wheatgrass are in addition sources of other valuable minerals (especially calcium, magnesium and potassium), vitamins and enzymes.

Magnesium
This natural antihistamine is often lacking in diets high in processed foods. It is also not absorbed by the body properly if it is eaten with too much sugar or foods high in fat.

Magnesium helps regulate body temperature and normalizes nerve action and muscle contraction. Whole grains, green leafy vegetables, soy beans, nuts and milk are the best sources of magnesium.

Vitamin B5 (pantothenic acid)
Food sources include whole grains, broad beans, egg yolk and liver. Too much alcohol, coffee, tea and stress increase the need for this vitamin. Possible symptoms of a Vitamin B5 deficiency include fatigue, fluid retention, sore feet, sleep disturbances, irritability and muscle cramps.

Vitamin B6 (pyridoxine)

Studies suggest that asthmatics may have a greater need for this vitamin than most people and further details of this are given on pages 105–6. Asthmatics should make an effort to eat a diet rich in Vitamin B6, even if they do not take supplements of it. Foods that have high B6 levels include whole-grain cereals, bananas, liver, avocado and lean meat. Vitamin B6 deficiency signs are low blood sugar, tiredness, depression, dermatitis and other skin problems, and susceptibility to infections.

Vitamin B12 (cobalamin)

Vitamin B12 reduces the effects of toxins and helps combat the effects of metabisulphites in those sensitive to them. Smoking, alcohol, diabetes and the overuse of laxatives increase the body's need for B12, which can be obtained from meat, liver, sardines, oysters, egg yolk and cheese.

Vitamin C

Another natural antihistamine (a substance that dampens down the inflammatory reaction), Vitamin C is also a mild antibiotic and is without doubt the most important vitamin for the treatment of respiratory ailments. Vitamin C protects us from colds, flu, sinus and similar complaints. It also appears to prevent asthma – see pages 103–5.

Rosehip syrup has the richest content of Vitamin C of all known foods, with an average of 520 mg per 100 g. Black currants, cranberries, parsley, horseradish, turnip, cabbage, strawberries, grapefruit, pineapple, tomatoes and watercress are also rich in Vitamin C, although it is found to some extent in all fresh fruits and vegetables.

Vitamin E (tocopherol)

Essential for healing, muscle, nerve and blood maintenance, Vitamin E also stabilises cell membranes. It has been recognised as an antioxidant, protecting vulnerable chemicals in the body from being destroyed by free radicals. It protects cells of the body from damage by environmental pollution.

Vitamin E is found in many foods, but wheat germ, almonds and vegetable oils are particularly rich in it.

Zinc

Zinc is a part of many enzymes in the body and is needed for the formation of proteins and insulin. It is also an all-round valuable nutrient for the body's immune system. It stabilizes the blood and maintains the acid/alkaline balance of the body.

Zinc helps the immune system by clearing out certain toxic metals like cadmium and lead, absorbed by our bodies from car exhaust fumes. Zinc is therefore an essential mineral for asthmatics who are affected by fumes and air pollutants. A shortage of zinc can appreciably lower the body's immune system. Up to 3 mg of zinc can be lost every day through sweating. Long-term use of laxatives, a diet excessively high in fiber, calcium or iron levels can also create a zinc deficiency; white marks on the finger nails are a common sign of zinc deficiency.

Dairy products, liver, meat, chicken, fish, oysters, green leafy vegetables and whole-grain bread all contain zinc, although much is lost if food is processed. ·

Seaweed or kelp

Seaweed is a special food, for it contains a wide range of valuable minerals. Particularly high in calcium, iodine, zinc, potassium, magnesium and selenium, seaweed is also very rich in Vitamin C – an additional bonus for someone with asthma. Seaweed stimulates the immune system and in the past folk medicine used it to treat respiratory and gastrointestinal problems. Seaweed has also been shown to lower cholesterol and blood pressure and to maintain balanced thyroid activity. Harvested from the sea bed, seaweed has added minerals not usually associated with "earthly" produce.

Japanese cuisine uses seaweed extensively, but Western cooking is not as adventurous. Rather than being served as a vegetable, or in sheets of *nori* wrapping sushi, we are more likely to encounter seaweed in powdered form or incorporated in prepared foods. The type of seaweed called carrageen is much used as a substitute for gelatin and is added to many convenience foods. Kelp is also used in a diverse collection of foods, including ice cream, salad dressings and desserts.

Supplementing Your Diet

The substances needed by the human body to grow and be healthy are contained in the food we eat, the liquids we drink and the air we breathe. However, it is a widely held belief by naturopaths, nutritionists and dietitians that a high proportion of people today are in fact suffering from deficiencies of one kind or another and that this is possibly the greatest threat we face to our health and longevity.

Many people still believe that eating a well-balanced diet will provide all the vitamins, minerals and enzymes necessary for good health. In ideal circumstances this is the case, but in reality a well-balanced diet is usually found in books and rarely on the table. Soil depletion, food processing, chemical additives, pesticide residues, toxic emissions, stress, emotional trauma and the overuse of drugs all increase our need for additional micronutrients to ensure a healthy life.

This need for added nutrients is much greater today than it was in past generations. Today's crops tend to be grown on mineral-depleted soils using artificial fertilizers, then manufactured with an eye towards appearance and processed to have a long shelf-life. During manufacture, many foods are refined to such a degree that most of their nutritional value is lost.

Your key to good health is a strong immune system and this requires plenty of nutrients. Although we have given details above of foods that are rich in particular vitamins and minerals, you may find that an optimum level of these substances can be maintained most effectively through supplementation. Supplements that contain a variety of ingredients are available in liquid, tablet or powder form from health food stores and pharmacies, and the recommended daily dosage is usually supplied with the particular product. If in doubt about what supplements would do you the most good, consult a practitioner.

Minerals

It is the function of minerals to build basic cell substances, and each cell needs specific minerals for the body's chemistry to work properly. There are about 25 minerals essential for good health.

Too little in the diet, or poor absorption by the body, can lead to serious deficiencies of them.

Calcium and phosphorus are present in the body in greater amounts than other minerals. Calcium is found mostly in bones and teeth and makes up about two per cent of body weight – nearly 1.5 kg – of a healthy, 70 kg adult. Phosphorus, again mostly in bones and teeth, makes up about 1.5 per cent of body weight and the total body content of this mineral is replaced every three years.

Of the other major minerals, iron forms only 0.006 per cent of the body yet is critical for life as it is contained in the hemo-globin of the red blood cells. Other vital minerals are sodium and potassium. Trace elements such as chromium, cobalt, copper, fluorine, iodine, manganese, molybdenum, selenium, sulphur and zinc are present in the body in smaller quantities but are still needed in minute amounts.

Age and circumstance govern the amount of minerals a body requires. For instance, although children usually need less min-erals than adults, growing children (under 17 years) need more calcium; women require more iron than men and pregnant women and nursing mothers need additional iron and calcium.

The combination of mineral sources in a single meal, or the form the mineral is combined in, can affect the way the body absorbs it. For example, the uptake of iron is enhanced if it is eaten with Vitamin C, whereas the tannin in tea reduces uptake. The absorption of several minerals including calcium and zinc is reduced by too much bran in the diet, and if the body is deficient in Vitamin D calcium will not be absorbed properly. A greater proportion of iron is absorbed from food if it is eaten in meat rather than contained in fresh green vegetables.

Of course, not all minerals are good for you in large quan-tities. For instance, too much salt (sodium chloride) in the diet causes high blood pressure in some people. Selenium and boron are other minerals where there is evidence that excess is not good for the health.

Asthma, sinus problems and catarrh can be the result of a mineral deficiency, particularly zinc, and supplementing the diet can bridge the deficit. Zinc has potent antiviral functions and stimulates the immune system. However, if you are considering a zinc supplement, you will also need more Vitamin A.

It is also common for asthmatics to have below normal red blood cell counts, that is, anemia. Symptoms include constant tiredness, palpitations, severe headaches, tachycardia (racing heartbeat), loss of appetite, shortness of breath, dizziness and ringing in the ears. Anemia is treated with extra iron and Vitamin B12. Selenium is sometimes suggested also, but only in minimal doses on a short-term basis.

Apple cider vinegar, nature's own drug-free anti-inflammatory, is rich in potassium, phosphorus and calcium, with lesser amounts of iron, chlorine, sodium, magnesium, sulphur, silicon and other trace minerals. This natural storehouse of good nutrients also contains amino acids, pectin and beta-carotene. Research centers and scientific studies around the world praise the preventive and curative powers of apple cider vinegar and we recommend that all asthmatics take a daily spoonful of it.

A good all-round remedy for bronchial conditions, including asthma, is a mixture of equal parts of lemon juice, honey and apple cider vinegar. Melt the honey in a small amount of hot water before mixing in the apple cider vinegar and lemon juice. You can make up enough for a few days and store it in the refrigerator. An effective dose when suffering from bronchial ailments is one tablespoon three times a day for adults, or one teaspoon three times a day for children. The honey will ease the throat, the apple cider vinegar will help reduce inflammation and the lemon juice provides Vitamin C.

If you are taking mineral supplements in a natural form they will not normally interfere with other treatments. They are compatible with herbs, vitamins and orthodox medication. You can also take them as part of a complete supplement. (See pages 106–7.)

You may also come across Schuessler tissue salts or biochemic mineral salts. These are not mineral supplements, but are homeopathic medicines and are described further in Chapter 9.

Vitamins

The Latin derivation of the word vitamin is from **vita**, meaning "life." Vitamins are substances necessary for life, being essential for growth and health. Our bodies are under constant pressure with today's stressful demands, and require masses of energy to maintain often far too busy lifestyles.

How can vitamins help? They work in various ways. They are involved in turning the food we eat into energy; they help build up specific parts of the body, especially the red blood cells, enzymes and fatty acids; they play an important role in growth of bones, teeth, blood vessels, and maintaining these (plus the skin and mucous membranes of the body) in good health. Some vitamins have antioxidant roles, which means they protect vulnerable fatty acids from being destroyed by free radicals in the body. Free radicals are formed by oxidation processes (natural chemical reactions) and by radiation. Although you may not be familiar with the word oxidation, you will recognize it: it's what happens when you cut open an apple or potato and the flesh turns brown. The fatty acids at risk in the body are found in the cell walls and nerve coverings, so ingesting plenty of antioxidants will help your body perform much better overall. Finally, of course, vitamins play an essential role in boosting the immune system and so increase the body's resistance to infection.

Do you need extra vitamins? Since asthmatics have generally poorer, or more stressed, immune systems than nonasthmatics, and frequently have overstimulated mucous membranes, you do need to ensure that your vitamin intake is sufficient to **heal**, not just to keep the status quo. Review your diet and take a long hard look at just what your body is absorbing. Are you getting enough vitamins and nutrients? Are they the right ones for you? Will they help your asthma?

While it may be argued that with a balanced diet it is unnecessary to take supplementary vitamins, the generally poor nutritional quality of the average diet, plus ignorance about vitamin-rich ingredients, combine to produce a deficiency of vitamins in most people. So a lot of the population would benefit from supplementing their food.

You don't have to worry about exactly how much you need, either, as large amounts of vitamins taken in a natural form are not generally harmful and will be excreted by the body if in excess. Very few people take into consideration the harm done to the body when they consume large amounts of tobacco, alcohol, chocolates, sugar and the like. Why then do people object to taking "too many vitamins"?

Which Vitamins?

Vitamins all play their parts in the body. A deficiency of Vitamin A will increase susceptibility to infection, as will deficiency of Vitamin D. Vitamin E protects the mucous membranes and can increase resistance to bacterial and yeast infections. Vitamins B6 and B5 stimulate the immune system; a vitamin B6 deficiency is associated with depletion of white blood cells in the thymus, spleen and lymph nodes and lowered antibody production. Combinations of various vitamins with omega 3 and omega 6 oils regulate inflammatory reactions in the body.

Vitamins A and D also improve the digestive system, stimulate bowel function and help rid the body of any build-up of toxic matter. These vitamins are easily absorbed in the form of cod liver oil. Cod liver oil, along with castor oil, was claimed in the past to "help oil the joints," and will no doubt conjure up some childhood memories for the more mature readers of this book. They were cure-alls used by mothers earlier this century. Many a child trying to avoid going to school by claiming they "weren't feeling well" was soon sent scurrying out the door by the threat of a "dose of oil to fix you up." Today, cod liver oil is available in convenient and more digestible capsules or tablets.

Vitamin C and Vitamin B6 are the two vitamins that have the most easily demonstrated effects on asthma, and we will cover these in greater detail below. For the other vitamins we suggest taking a complete supplement (see pages 106–7).

VITAMIN C

Vitamin C has been recognized as a powerful and useful part of the diet for hundreds of years, since it was first associated with preventing scurvy in sailors. It is without doubt the most important of the vitamins required for anyone who suffers from any respiratory complaint, including asthma. Dr. Linus Pauling, the Nobel prize winner, is most emphatic in his book *Vitamin C and the Common Cold* about the need to take 2000–3000 mg (2–3 g) of Vitamin C per day for bronchial and respiratory conditions.

Pauling concentrated on the effect of large doses of Vitamin C on the cold virus, but investigations have revealed that people receiving 100–200 mg Vitamin C per day show a decrease in the incidence of other conditions, for example, asthma, glandular fever, laryngitis and chronic fatigue syndrome.

In Nigeria, where asthmatic symptoms have been shown to be worse during the wet season, a trial was carried out using Vitamin C. The asthmatics were divided into two groups, and 1000 mg (1 g) of Vitamin C was given daily to one group of asthmatics and a placebo to the control group. Symptoms decreased in 75 per cent of those who took the Vitamin C. When the group stopped taking Vitamin C their asthma attacks returned to their previous rate. It is not clear, however, whether the drop in asthma symptoms was due to a drop in respiratory viruses as a result of taking the vitamin (colds are frequently a trigger for asthma) or whether the Vitamin C was preventing asthma by dampening the allergic or inflammatory response.

Another study was conducted by Dr. Schachter at Yale University, focusing on the ability of Vitamin C to relieve exercise-induced asthma. Those in the study took 500 mg of Vitamin C before exercise and it was found that following the exercise the severity of their bronchospasms was lessened significantly. Dr. Schachter made it clear in his results that Vitamin C was by no means the most effective agent that could be used for reducing bronchospasm, but it is a beneficial natural remedy with limited and minor side effects.

Scientific studies may provide evidence in favor of Vitamin C, but there is also a huge weight of anecdotal evidence from the public. Many people take Vitamin C supplements and say how the number of colds and bouts of flu they catch have lessened since taking Vitamin C. Most of these will be taking 1000–2000 mg a day, and are reluctant to reduce this amount because they feel it is doing them so much good.

Because Vitamin C is not stored in the body, an adequate amount of Vitamin C must be taken daily. To consume the 2000 mg that Pauling recommends someone would need to eat about 30 oranges a day, but there are supplements that can be taken easily. An economical one is ascorbic acid, which can be bought in powder form and mixed with orange juice. Half a teaspoon is approximately 2000 mg. You can't overdose on Vitamin C, as any excess will be eliminated.

Although overdosing is not dangerous, it can have unpleasant side-effects, and it is important to build up your intake of

Vitamin C slowly. Reported side effects include diarrhea, discoloration of urine and a burning sensation when it is being passed. If this happens, reduce the amount of Vitamin C until your body becomes accustomed to it. We suggest you begin supplementing with only a pinch or so of ascorbic acid powder, building up to a quarter to half a teaspoon daily.

If you don't want to take supplements, rosehip syrup is the richest food source of Vitamin C, with an average of 520 mg per 100 g. Black currants, parsley, horseradish, turnip, cabbage, strawberries, grapefruit, pineapple, tomatoes and watercress, along with most fresh fruits and vegetables, are also rich in it.

A simple and inexpensive test is now available on the market to measure the level of Vitamin C in your body, using a urinary ascorbate stick, and there are other uncomplicated tests that can be carried out to measure your Vitamin C. If your reading is low, it is in your interest to increase your intake.

Smoking is one of the worst things an asthmatic can do, as it directly takes pollutants and allergic triggers into the sensitive airways. However, it is not so widely known that cigarette smoking uses up Vitamin C in the body. Levels of the vitamin have been measured in smokers and it has been shown that one cigarette can use up to 25 mg of Vitamin C. It is therefore doubly important that asthmatics who smoke supplement their diet with Vitamin C. Obviously the best solution would be to stop smoking altogether, and you will find suggestions to help you do so in Chapter 15.

VITAMIN B6

Researchers studying the effects of Vitamin B6 on anemic patients discovered that it was also beneficial to asthma. The study, which was led by Clayton L. Natta, M.D., associate professor of medicine at Columbia University, found that the patients were reporting improvement in their asthma symptoms when they took 50 mg of B6 daily. Further studies have since been conducted on asthmatics, which have supported the effectiveness of B6.

J. Collip, M.D., of the Department of Pediatrics at the Nassau County N.Y. Medical Center, undertook a rigorous scientific study with 76 young patients aged 2–16 years. Without going into specific details of this study, it was found that children taking

200 mg of Vitamin B6 daily experienced less frequent asthma attacks, less wheezing, less tightness in the chest and less breathing difficulties. As a result of taking Vitamin B6 less medication was also necessary. The study concluded that pyridoxine B6 therapy may be useful in reducing the severity of asthma, in children in particular.

Studies at the University of California, Los Angeles, also suggest that Vitamin B6 is beneficial for asthmatics and that 100 mg should be taken three times daily. It may, however, be more useful to take the Vitamin B6 incorporated with the full B complex, as this is believed to improve assimilation.

A word of warning: megadoses of B6 can be toxic and are not recommended. For an adult 50 mg is known to be a safe dose. If you wish to take more than this amount you should consult a practitioner first.

BIOFLAVONOIDS (VITAMIN P)

Bioflavonoids reduce inflammation and tissue swelling. Sometimes they are known as Vitamin P, and rutin is the most common type of bioflavonoid. Naturopaths usually recommend bioflavonoid supplements for people with asthma. The effect of a bioflavonoid supplement is enhanced when combined with Vitamin C. Although found in the rind, and to some extent, the juice and pulp of citrus fruits, Vitamin P is also contained in grapes, plums, black currants, cherries and rosehips and the skin of bright-colored vegetables like carrots. However, these sources do not generally provide sufficient bioflavonoids in the daily diet to have an effect on asthma.

The Right Vitamin and Mineral Supplement

The best combination for asthmatics or respiratory condition sufferers is at least two multivitamin capsules daily, containing in total about:

VITAMIN A 10 000 IU	BIOTIN 5 mg
VITAMIN D 1000 IU	BETA-CAROTENE 3 mg
VITAMIN B1 10 mg	CALCIUM 10 mg
VITAMIN B2 10 mg	MAGNESIUM 10 mg

VITAMIN B6 5 mg	IRON 8.25 mg
VITAMIN B12 5 mg	MANGANESE 0.65 mg
VITAMIN C 100 mg	COPPER 0.1 mg
VITAMIN E 10 mg	ZINC 0.8 mg
NIACINAMIDE 30 mg	POTASSIUM 0.95 mg
CALCIUM PANTOTHENATE 10 mg	IODINE 3 mg
INOSITOL 15 mg	PHOSPHORUS 6.5 mg
FOLATE 1 mg	

This broad vitamin and mineral intake can be found in a variety of proprietary vitamin supplements, so should be easy for you to take. It doesn't quite cover everything an asthmatic requires, though, so we recommend that **in addition** you should take extra Vitamin A and Vitamin D, preferably in the natural and concentrated form of a cod liver oil capsule, along with 2000–2500 mg of Vitamin C using ascorbate acid or rosehip juice (see advice above on building up the dose slowly).

Vitamin E in the form of a spoonful of wheat germ daily is also good for asthmatics and if Vitamin P (bioflavonoids) improves your asthma you should add it to your daily supplement.

The quantities recommended for supplementation are for adults only. Children's supplements should be half of these, and you should not supplement infants without practitioner advice.

Other Dietary Supplements

Of course, vitamin and mineral supplements are only a small part of the industry that promotes dietary supplements of all kinds. Negotiating your way through the maze of information about herbs, amino acids, enzymes and other unfamiliar nutrients, and working out what might be useful for you, is a daunting task – a bit like going on a cross-country trek with a myriad of signposts pointing in different directions. It can be overwhelming. You can probably imagine your home being swamped with little bottles, and spending most of your time swallowing endless pills. Relax: it doesn't have to be like this!

Your wisest course of action before launching into a sea of

supplements would be to consult a naturopath, herbalist or nutritionist who can accurately assess your health, diet and lifestyle and identify your supplement needs. By consulting an expert you will also learn about recommended dosages and eliminate the possibility of overloading your body or wasting your money on too many of the wrong supplements. Some supplements have to be introduced gradually, some may conflict with others and could defeat the purpose of optimum nutritional benefit.

However, if you choose to "do it yourself," do investigate the content and nutrient value of supplements. Avoid any where the ingredients contain artificial colorings or preservatives. You will sometimes see the labels list "chelated" minerals – these are more readily digestible than ordinary minerals and so absorbed better.

Try a course of one particular supplement at a time. Don't start on a cocktail of pills otherwise you may never know just which one is really doing you good. Most suppliers are diligent in eliminating as many possible allergenic substances from their products but some can contain impurities.

Bargain products should be considered with caution. There is usually a reason why they are so cheap – they are not ultimately a bargain if quality is lacking. Rely on reputable brands and take advice from registered practitioners with approved qualifications.

When you begin to introduce supplements to your diet, be sure to also drink a liter or more of water a day. This will maintain adequate kidney function. After a few weeks see what happens: if the supplement is providing nutrients generally lacking in your diet your health will improve, you will be invigorated, you will achieve that wonderful feeling of being well!

There are many conveniently packaged food supplements and enzyme-rich organic superfoods being sold in health food stores. Powder formulas can be simply mixed with milk, water or juice, and biscuits or cookies provide a combination of many nutrients. These can easily be assimilated into your regular diet. The biscuits or cookies can be your snack between meals, and the powder combinations can be your morning or afternoon drinks. Multinutrient capsules and tablets which contain most vitamins, proteins, amino acids and minerals from a natural source, such as spiruliten (spirulina), also make adequate dietary supplements that are convenient and easy to take.

The following nutrient supplements are particularly suitable for anyone with asthma or respiratory disorders.

SPIRULINA AND CHLORELLA
Rich in chlorophyll, minerals, vitamins and a great source of protein, chlorella and spirulina regulate cholesterol, promote anti-viral action and stimulate the immune system. The ancient Aztecs called spirulina the 'sacred power plant,' and believed it was endowed with the energy of the sun and had remarkable energizing and rejuvenating properties.

Spirulina is derived from fresh-water algae and contains a complex abundance of enzymes, vitamins, minerals, trace elements and amino acids and other biochemicals. It is now grown in aqua farms.

EVENING PRIMROSE OIL
The secret behind the oil of this unassuming flower is its gamma-linoleic acid (GLA) content, a substance that is extremely valuable to the body. Most vegetable oils contain linoleic acid, which the body has to convert into GLA before use; some people who are atopic may be unable to convert linoleic acid into GLA. They are thought to be deficient in a particular enzyme that is needed for the conversion process.

GLA is used by the body to produce a hormone-like anti-inflammatory substance – a prostaglandin – which is capable of stimulating particular cells in the immune system. It is believed that asthma sufferers have stressed immune responses, which may be helped by GLA.

Experiments have also shown that GLA assists greatly in reducing cholesterol and triglyceride levels, further cleansing the body and thereby aiding asthma. Of course, evening primrose oil is often prescribed for PMS and eczema too.

ROYAL JELLY
This ancient Chinese food of nature is made by bees; it is the special food fed to the larvae who will grow up to be queens rather than workers. Royal jelly has been used for centuries to ward off disease: Hippocrates is said to have mentioned it in his teachings in the fourth century BC. Royal jelly is not used as a

drug to combat any particular disease, but rather as a health-giving supplement.

Royal jelly contains numerous trace elements, mainly copper, calcium, iron and silica, which are of paramount importance to the body's immune system. Royal jelly is said to contain virtually every nutritional element needed for a healthy diet and to optimize resistance against asthma and respiratory disorders. Recently, however, some side effects have been recorded in connection with the pollen in royal jelly. Although evidence is not yet clear, it appears that some people can have severe allergic reactions to it and several deaths have been reported. Asthmatics tend to be allergic. Be **extremely** cautious if considering royal jelly as a supplement and introduce it slowly.

Royal jelly is mainly prepared in a liquid form within a small capsule and taken on a daily basis.

Food Allergies and Additives

Asthma can be triggered by what you eat, so be careful, and be aware of the ingredients in your food.

Why do substances cause allergy, and asthma, in some people, but others are unharmed by eating them? We don't have any real answer yet, as every allergic substance may be acting in a different way. However, it appears that a major factor contributing to allergic asthma is an impaired immune system.

We all face difficulties in assessing, treating and helping our health problems, but for those with problems associated with diet, eating – which should be one of life's pleasures – can become constantly stressful. Nevertheless, don't be discouraged. Believe in the healing power of Nature and find her key to unlocking the door to a healthier, asthma-free life.

Only you, the asthmatic, can determine precisely what food, or additive, affects you. It is not uncommon for asthmatics to be allergic to a number of different foods. Asthma can be triggered by eating nuts like peanuts, cashews or walnuts, and dairy produce, eggs and yeast products. Fish, especially seafood, tomatoes and spices are also known triggers for some people. Anything manufactured that contains additives is of course suspect: cookies, potato chips, cakes, carbonated drinks, cordials and ice cream may all cause asthma. You can probably add your own triggers to this list.

Some infant milk preparations contain vegetable oil derived from peanuts, and an article in the *Lancet* of 29 May 1993 suggested this is possibly responsible for the increased incidence among children of an allergic sensitivity to peanuts.

Yeast products, too, should be avoided by chronic asthmatics, as a substance known to cause excessive mucus secretion, constriction of airways and activation of inflammatory cells (all part of asthmatic reactions) is found in yeast. Yeast is a good source of many vitamins, but you may have to find an alternative in your diet.

Supermarket convenience foods are usually heavily refined, with preservatives and artificial colorings being added. The preparation also leads to loss of micronutrients, particularly vitamins B1, B2, B3, C, E and zinc. The food processing industry has contributed to the increase in asthma in today's society, as well as to other diseases of our time like diverticulitis, gall stones, heart disease, varicose veins, diabetes and constipation, among many others. There is also evidence that hyperactivity in children is often related to their diet.

If you don't know exactly what is causing your asthma but suspect it is caused by a food, start a food diary. List everything you eat. When you have an attack look at the diary and see if you can link any particular food to previous asthma attacks. Elimination diets, where you eat only a few items and gradually introduce those you suspect may be causing problems, can identify asthma-causing foods, but they should only be carried out under practitioner supervision. Elimination diets are not in general suitable for children.

SODIUM METABISULPHITE

Sodium metabisulphite is an additive used to prevent bacteria growing in foods, preserve colors of canned and prepared foods and retain Vitamin C. It is added to drinks including alcohol and fruit juices, toppings, salad dressings, flavorings, jams, dried fruits and vegetables, sausages, "fresh" shrimp and fruit yogurt. It has been shown to have strong links to childhood asthma, especially where the child also has a folic acid deficiency.

A recent study in a Sydney hospital revealed that up to 65

per cent of asthmatics they treated were so sensitive to sodium metabisulphite that it provoked an asthma attack shortly after they ate it. So nearly two out of every three asthmatics could trigger an attack by eating common foods like tinned soup, pickles, sausages, snack foods, dried fruit, dehydrated potatoes, commercial fruit juices and the like.

TARTRAZINE

Most children (and many adults) like to eat and drink foods containing the common additive tartrazine. It turns up everywhere – in syrups, toppings, sauces, soft drinks, cordials, frozen sweets, confectionery, snack foods, jellies, cookies, puddings and is also used to color medicines yellow, green or orange!

Identifying Additives

Food companies sometimes seem to the outsider to be playing God with our health and our lives because of their use of additives, preservatives and artificial colorings. However, consumers have some help, as there are now government guidelines controlling food labelling. All ingredients in a manufactured food must be listed on the label or packaging somewhere in descending order by weight. For those of us who are asthmatic and allergic to certain additives, or who are following a restricted diet, knowledge of the ingredients is vital.

The additives are usually listed on the food by name. Artificial colors are given FD&C numbers by the Food and Drug Administration.

Here are some additives that have been linked to asthma:

Tartrazine	Sulphur dioxide
Sunset yellow FCF	Sodium sulphite
Amaranth	Sodium bisulphite
Erythrosine	Sodium metabisulphite
Brilliant blue FCF	Potassium metabisulphite
Benzoic acid	Butylated hydroxyanisole BHA
Sodium benzoate	Butylated hydroxytoluene BHT
Potassium benzoate	Monosodium glutamate
Calcium benzoate	

Improve Your Diet!

Unfortunately, in today's world the food we choose to eat is often based on cost or convenience rather than on its nutritional value. The most effective ways to treat your asthmatic condition are to revitalize your immune system with good nutrition, decrease the toxins in your body, avoid allergy triggers and conditions and exercise regularly. Have a balanced diet including lots of fruit and vegetables, grown chemical-free if possible, and increase the range of vitamins, minerals and herbs you eat.

Remember, the decision is yours. Good health is a choice – how good do you want to feel? Changing or improving your diet is a positive step in the right direction. If you eliminate asthma-triggering preservatives and additives from your diet, eat nutrition-loaded foods and increase your fluid intake, you will feel better. You will be more inclined to want to exercise and learn breathing techniques to manage your asthma. Before long your energy levels will increase, the stress of asthma will be eased, you will feel relaxed and able to cope with your condition. Thriving – not just surviving!

Juices

Juices extracted from plants, fruits, vegetables or herbs are extremely rich in vitamins, natural sugars, minerals, enzymes and trace elements. Very few other foods are as good for us as the raw juices of fruits or vegetables.

They are assimilated directly from the stomach into the bloodstream without undue strain on the digestive system. They aid the body in purifying the blood, help in neutralizing waste products, assist in building new tissue and have a revitalizing and rejuvenating effect on the body's organs and glands.

Raw fruit and vegetables have a particularly high Vitamin C content, which oxygenates the blood, destroys foreign bacteria, clears cholesterol, builds resistance to disease, speeds up the healing process and is a powerful boost to the immune system. High doses of Vitamin C protect us against the common cold, asthma and respiratory conditions.

Many juicing experts advise that you should not mix

vegetable and fruit juices as it can cause assimilation and digestive difficulties. Although best taken on their own, various fruit juices can be combined, for example orange and pineapple, apple and prune juices. Take care with watermelon and mango – some people are allergic to them.

Supermarket shelves overflow with a mouthwatering assortment of juices but very few of them can be considered fresh and contain too many additives or preservatives to be of much nutritional value. Read the labels carefully. The best way to consume healthy juices is to make them yourself: you can have freshly prepared fruit or vegetable juices on tap and create your own taste sensations if you buy a juice extractor. It will probably become the most used appliance in your kitchen.

Adopt the daily habit of drinking a glass of fruit or vegetable juice before breakfast and add to this a half to one teaspoon (1500-2500 mg) of ascorbic acid (Vitamin C). This is also a great time to take your multi-vitamin capsule and any other supplements that are benefiting you.

If you find cold vegetable juices unpalatable there are many juices which can be served hot as soups (but don't boil away the goodness from them). An equal blend of vegetables grown above and below the ground makes a delicious and healthy mix to include in your diet. Make the most of locally grown, preferably organic, vegetables when they are in season and reasonably priced. In the winter, thick vegetable soup and fresh bread makes a hearty, nutritious meal for the whole family.

Mono-Diet

Mono-diets are not suitable for children.

The human body functions 24 hours a day, seven days a week, 365 days a year. Occasionally it needs to be given a rest. One of the most effective ways to give your body a holiday is with a three-day mono-diet. It puts the digestive organs into go-slow mode. The liver, gall bladder, stomach, pancreas and intestines work continuously and a mono-diet gives them time to regroup.

Nature sometimes forces a compulsory rest on us by reducing our taste for food and depressing our appetite. When we get a cold or other illness, or sometimes when we just feel run down, we don't feel like eating much. It is possible for a person to exist without food for quite a long period of time – consider hunger strikers, who can last for weeks without eating – but not fluids. Liquid is essential for sustenance and survival. A mono-diet involves just taking liquid.

Throughout history many different cultures have encouraged fasting in the belief that it is good for moral, spiritual and physical well-being. However, most people are reluctant to attempt a program that requires a great deal of discipline, determination and willpower, unless they seriously want to correct their dietary habits.

A mono-diet for only three days is short enough to be able to contemplate without fear of failure, and will establish a foundation on which you can build a new and improved eating regimen. But don't just rush in and think "I'll start today." **Do not attempt to fast unless you are asthma-free and in good health**, nor if you have a busy work or exercise schedule. Choose a time when you have no social engagements and are able to rest, such as a long weekend. It is also advisable to consult your health practitioner to check that your body can cope with the sudden change to its metabolism.

Your only intake for three days will be the freshly squeezed juice of a single fruit or vegetable, such as orange, apple, grapefruit, carrot, celery or cabbage. You can use your own juice extractor or purchase prepared pure, additive-free juices from health food stores.

Only **one** type of juice should be consumed and it is important that the mono-diet last for three whole days. It will not be easy, especially on the second day when symptoms of nausea, headache and giddiness may occur, but these feelings will probably pass with rest. The symptoms are caused by the readjustment the body's metabolism must make, especially when withdrawing from the likes of tea or coffee. (Smokers and excessive drinkers who have kicked the habit know all about withdrawal symptoms.) If you have a very bad headache, then you can take a limited amount of tea or coffee – or whatever addictive element you have gone without – to alleviate it.

On the third day there will be a marked improvement in how you feel, and any hunger will have lessened. You will feel better – probably better than you have for years. Once you have completed the three days, break the fast slowly by eating the fruit or vegetable of the juice that you have been drinking. So if you chose orange juice, eat an orange. After the first meal you can gradually introduce different varieties of fruit or vegetables, before progressing to salad-type meals over a period of days. It will then be relatively easy to alter your previous eating habits, including many more fruit and vegetables. Create and follow a sensible eating plan for yourself to keep your body on track.

Sometimes our hectic lifestyle prevents us from maintaining a balanced diet and our body suffers. If, or when, things "get away" from you, do the three-day mono-diet again, provided at least 28 days have elapsed since the previous mono-diet.

For some people such a program will require a great deal of discipline, but like most things which demand effort, it will have its rewards. The old saying, "No pain, no gain," certainly applies here.

NATURAL REMEDIES

"It is not enough for man to be his creator for health and long life. He should also use his intelligence to discover and bring to light the treasures graciously hidden by God in Nature as a means of healing the ills of his human life." Sebastian Kneipp (1821–97)

The Western world looks after the sick, and doctors are paid for making ill patients better. But is this the most efficient way to keep people healthy? In some Eastern countries, the approach is reversed. The focus is on preventive care and healers are paid for keeping people well. When their "patients" do become ill, it is still their responsibility to care for them and restore them to good health. As their financial reward is based on the number of healthy people in their care, these healers concentrate on the overall well-being of a person and utilize as many natural treatments as possible to keep them well.

One can't help but ask whether the general health of the Western world would also be improved if this concept was adopted. If medical practitioners applied their knowledge to preventing illness, and were justly rewarded for their success, perhaps they would be working harder to recommend improvements to our lifestyles and nutrition. They might consider environmental factors affecting our health, and try natural methods instead of drugs as the answer to all our ills.

The world of medicine is similar to the world of politics. In democracies people demand a change of government when they are dissatisfied with the performance of the present one; and we believe that if there was sufficient demand – "people power" – pressuring orthodox medicine to provide alternative avenues to health, it would be motivated to change. Preventing illness is just as vital as curing illness and society today is seeking choices and guidance to improve health and secure a disease-free future.

If you want to explore the choices available to you, at present you have to consult alternative practitioners. There are a number of traditions of complementary therapies, and below we give an introduction to four that use remedies derived from the natural world around us – herbs, flowers, oils and minerals – and how they may be useful for people with asthma.

Herbal Medicine

Shen-nung was a Chinese emperor born more than 5000 years ago. Records indicate that he used plants medicinally; to treat bronchial and asthmatic problems he used ma-huang. In recent times it has been found that ma-huang contains ephedrine, a drug now frequently prescribed for asthma and pulmonary disorders.

So it is with many herbal medicines: they contain small but natural amounts of drugs that do have real effects on many conditions. Because they are obtained from plants, they do not just contain one ingredient, as a pharmaceutical drug will, but can have a number of active principles, and so may help the overall health of a patient, not just attacking the immediate symptoms.

Herbalism has a long history in many cultures, as well as China. Remedies prepared from various plants were used in ancient Greek and Egyptian civilizations. It appears that respiratory ailments were treated by the Greeks with herbs such as mint, garlic, cloves and myrrh. Nicholas Culpeper, the famous seventeenth-century English astronomer and physician, now recognized as the father of modern Western herbalism, was a strong advocate of natural remedies. He encouraged people to

follow a natural lifestyle, and emphasized the benefits of botan-
ical medicine. His legacy to future generations was a vast collection of herbal remedies which are as valuable today as they were
more than 300 years ago.

Modern technology has demonstrated that plants and herbs
contain invaluable properties and a great interest is now being
taken in their powers to heal. Herbal remedies are at present
enjoying a revival, with an increasing number of people insisting
on a more natural form of healing.

There is an enormous variety of plants from which herbal
remedies are derived. Generally speaking, herbs for medicinal
purposes are readily available. This was, of course, vital in the
days before the invention of the automobile, when the opportu-
nities for travel were limited. Medicine had to be accessible to
the population.

Herbs are seldom used singularly, herbalists preferring to
prescribe a number together. This is because they are often treating several symptoms, not just one. For instance, when someone
with asthma consults an herbalist he or she may be prescribed
herbs to cut down on mucus production, herbs to ease bronchospasms and coughing, and herbs to build up the immune
system – for, as we have seen, a strong and robust immune
system lessens the likelihood of severe asthma occurring.

Most herbal suppliers provide combination formulas developed specially for asthma, which contain a number of herbs.
Here is an example of the constituents of one: passionflower,
common thyme, grindelia, euphorbia, ascorbic acid, Vitamin A
acetate. Another recognized herbal mixture readily available contains proportions of horehound, euphorbia, senega, grindelia,
licorice and elecampane.

Horseradish and garlic tablets, available in odorless form, are
recommended to help eliminate excessive mucus. Some years ago
a common remedy for keeping breathing passages clear was to
wear a camphor block enclosed in a calico bag attached to
underclothes. Nowadays, not too many people would consider
wearing camphor but it does help free blocked airways while
sleeping. Camphor is dangerous if swallowed, should not be
handled directly and must be kept out of the reach of children.

There are a number of ways of preparing herbs for use. Different parts of the plants can also be used: bark, leaves, flowers

or roots. Herbal remedies can take the form of ointments, poultices, inhalations, teas, decoctions, tablets and tinctures.

There are large numbers of herbal teas available on supermarket shelves, but you can also make your own. Brewing or infusion times vary, but generally for tender plants such as basil, sage, mint, being steeped in boiling water for five minutes is sufficient, whereas tough herbs like coltsfoot or horehound need 10 minutes. A tea can be drunk or gargled, depending on the herb or symptom you are treating.

This book cannot attempt to give detailed information about all the complementary modalities it discusses, but there are plenty of books available that will give you instructions on making herbal remedies if you are interested. Specialist herb gardeners or nurseries and herbal nutritionists will give you more specific information. And of course you don't have to make your own remedies: health food shops carry prepared herbal medicines and formulas, as will any practicing herbalist. You should also consult an herbalist for further recommendations if the common herbal remedies for asthma do not improve your condition.

Some of the most common herbs used for the relief of asthma and bronchial conditions are: euphorbia, lobelia, garlic, eucalyptus, coltsfoot, senega, vervain, aloe, echinacea, hyssop, horehound, honeysuckle, sage, aniseed, chamomile, ginkgo, comfrey, fennel, thyme, valerian, licorice, passionflower and grindelia. We cannot cover all of them in detail, but here is more information about a number of them.

GARLIC

Well-known in the kitchen, there is more to the humble *Allium sativum* bulb than just folklore. Garlic has been used for centuries and has the reputation of being an herb of amazing medicinal and nutritional value. Garlic possesses antiviral, antibacterial and antihistamine properties and also boosts the immune system; all these mean it is extremely beneficial to people with asthma prone to respiratory complaints. It is also an effective expectorant.

Researchers have discovered that one medium garlic clove has an antibacterial action approximately equivalent to 100 000 units of penicillin (a dose of penicillin is in the region of 1 million units). Garlic also contains selenium, a valuable antioxidant.

Extensive international research has resulted in garlic being assessed as a potent, broad-spectrum antibiotic and microorganism inhibitor – which leaves little doubt that garlic has pharmacological and therapeutic properties.

Garlic is also an effective herb for conditions other than asthma. It is known to decrease cholesterol and triglyceride levels in the blood and lower blood pressure. It is used to treat cardiovascular disease, colds and viral infections, hay fever, digestive disorders, and fungal infections such as thrush. In the past it has been recommended against intestinal parasites.

Garlic is best taken in its natural form, chopped or crushed to be more readily digestible. For an infusion, simply place 4–6 cloves in a cup of cool water and leave for six hours before drinking. Add 1–20 ml of brandy to preserve the garlic and break down its concentration.

Note   Avoid giving garlic to children under five years of age. If you have a clotting disorder consult your doctor about acceptable medicinal levels.

Garlic's odor is noticeable and the taste is strong. As a result many people are not comfortable with eating large amounts of raw garlic, or drinking garlic tea. This drawback has been overcome by the development of odorless garlic capsules or tablets, although some herbalists feel that these are less effective than the fresh clove. Capsules are widely available at pharmacies and health food stores, where you may also find garlic combined with horseradish, which is one of the best safeguards against colds, influenza, asthma and respiratory problems.

ECHINACEA

An herb native to North America, echinacea is highly regarded as a traditional treatment for immune disorders and infections of the upper respiratory tract such as asthma, colds, flu, tonsillitis and catarrh. It is considered one of the most powerful alternative medicines because of its excellent antibiotic, antiviral and immune-system boosting properties. Echinacea helps contain infection and shortens the duration of coughs, colds and flus. It is therefore an ideal herb for asthmatics to take regularly.

Echinacea is widely available in a variety of forms: liquid formulas to relieve mucus buildup and coughs, easy-to-take soft gel capsules and tablets.

GINKGO BILOBA

The therapeutic uses of extracts from the ginkgo biloba, or maidenhair tree, are centuries old. It is a species that has probably been around for hundreds of millions of years, and is believed extinct in the wild. It has survived in Far Eastern temple gardens and is popular in city streets and parks. Ginkgo biloba extract from the seeds aids asthma and respiratory problems, while the leaves are believed to be more beneficial for blood flow and circulation. Most commonly used recently to slow the decline of age, ginkgo enhances the mental faculties and helps overcome fatigue, depression and anxiety. Ginkgo can be purchased as extracts, tablets and capsules.

GINSENG

Called the most gentle "queen of herbs" and an all-healing plant, ginseng is said to be the most enduring and energy-giving tonic known to man. The Chinese and Koreans have used the ginseng root for more than 5000 years. Despite many tests to which modern scientists have subjected ginseng, no ill effects have been demonstrated to result from taking it.

Ginseng has a strong influence on the immune system and contains substances that are similar to steroids (a type of hormone in the human body) and also Vitamins B1, B2, and D. Ginseng is therefore recognized as a useful treatment for asthma and respiratory disorders, especially chronic coughs which often accompany asthma, and it is also used for exhaustion, nervous disorders, tuberculosis and circulatory problems.

There are different types of ginseng: Chinese or Asian, Siberian and American. Studies have revealed that because of differing hormonal levels, Siberian ginseng is more effective for women and the Chinese/Asian ginseng for men. Ginseng is available in many forms including capsules, powders, herbal teas and even chewing gum!

LICORICE

Hippocrates extolled the virtues of licorice as an aid for asthma, throat and chest problems. The herb was known elsewhere in the world: the American Indians used licorice as tea, as a cough remedy and as a soothing elixir for the throat. It is used today for all kinds of chest complaints, including asthma, and it also

has anti-inflammatory properties, which makes it especially beneficial for asthmatics.

A most beneficial healing herb when used in moderation,
licorice can be harmful if used in large amounts and should not
be taken by people with high blood pressure problems or those
using digitoxin-based drugs. Because of its sweetness, licorice is
often used in combination to camouflage the taste of more bitter
herbs to make them more palatable. The unique taste of licorice
has made this herb a worldwide favorite. Be warned, though:
licorice candy does not contain herbal licorice and is **not**
beneficial for your health!

LOBELIA

This small, blue-flowered plant, native to North America, is
sometimes known as Indian tobacco and was used in the late
eighteenth century by European settlers for the treatment of
asthma and respiratory complaints. Lobelia, which is also called
the "asthma weed," owes its effectiveness to the alkaloid coveline,
a respiratory stimulant. In the case of whooping cough, croup,
asthma or bronchitis, it acts as an expectorant, loosening mucus
from the surfaces of the air passages and rapidly clearing them
and the lungs of sticky foreign matter.

Lobelia is a strong herb and should never be prepared from
home-grown plants. It is available in manufactured remedies from
pharmacies. Some over-the-counter antismoking preparations
and cough mixtures contain lobelia.

EUCALYPTUS

Eucalyptus is often used in herbal preparations for the treatment
of asthma, but as the essential oil is the part used in the remedy,
we have covered it under Aromatherapy, pages 136–7.

ALOE VERA

Known since the days of ancient civilization as "the first aid plant"
because of its miraculous healing properties, aloe vera is used
worldwide. Known primarily for its power to aid healing of
wounds and burns it is also used as a skin cleanser, antiseptic,
moisturizer, nutrient and antioxidant. It promotes cell growth,
which is why it speeds up healing. It improves digestive tract
function and is prescribed also to treat constipation. With its

anti-inflammatory and antibacterial properties, aloe vera juice also effectively eases coughs, and the steam from the gel can be inhaled to soothe bronchial congestion – both applications useful for asthmatics.

A wide variety of preparations are available, including juices, gels, ointments, creams, lotions and shampoos.

Obtaining herbs

You should consult a reputable herbal practitioner when seeking herbal remedies, but health food stores can often supply proprietary lines. There are books on herbal medicine that will also recommend specific remedies.

When you have established just which herbs are best for you, why not start your own herb garden? Small windowbox planters or pots are all you need. Not only will you enjoy watching something grow but you will also have the wonderful aroma of fresh herbs wafting into your home. You can take time to "smell the herbs" and include them naturally in your cooking.

Homeopathy

Homeopathy is derived from the Greek words **homoios** meaning "like" and **pathos** meaning "suffering." It is a method of treating the sick based on the law "Similia similibus curantur," which translates loosely as "like being treated with like."

Homeopathy was developed by a German medical practitioner, Dr. Samuel Hahnemann, at the end of the eighteenth century. Dr. Hahnemann, like many scholars of his time, was very innovative and prepared to challenge orthodox medicine. He formulated the theory, based on his observations, that symptoms could be treated by taking tiny amounts of substances that would produce the **same symptoms** as the disease if taken in larger quantities. Since then homeopathic practitioners have been successfully healing the sick with little alteration from Dr. Hahnemann's original principles. Homeopathy, a safe, scientific and logical method for the treatment of sickness, has stood the test of time.

Homeopathy is believed to work because the remedies stimulate the immune system to fight the particular symptom pattern. It therefore helps the body heal itself. The remedies are given in very diluted forms, at such low concentrations that there is sometimes hardly a trace of the substance the remedy was originally made from. As a result orthodox medicine has not accepted homeopathy, arguing that the remedies have no active drugs in them, so can only be working as placebos. Homeopaths point to their success rate in treating disease (sometimes higher than for orthodox medical methods – for instance in the European cholera epidemic of 1854) as evidence that homeopathy works.

The homeopathic physician seeks to correct a disorder by treating the patient through the symptoms, not the symptoms themselves. This requires the homeopath to study the individual patient carefully. As the key to taking the right remedy is assessing the individual, especially in chronic conditions, it is essential to consult a homeopathic physician.

The symptoms on which a homeopathic prescription is based are not necessarily the symptoms of the disease, but the way the individual patient experiences the symptoms. The symptoms may even have no obvious connection with the disease. The most important groups of symptoms the homeopath looks at are mental, emotional, fears, cravings and aversions. Other symptoms include reactions to the weather and external conditions, the effects of heat and cold, lifestyle and work-related pressures, and so on.

Thus for asthma three patients who complain respectively of asthma with nausea and vomiting, asthma with muscle spasm, or asthma that is worst on waking, will be given three different remedies. Remedies most often used for asthma and acute congestion are aconite, arsenicum, sambucus, blatta, cuprum met, bryonia, belladonna, drosera, ignatia, pulsatilla, tuberculinum, ipecac and sulphur. Tissue salts (see overleaf) may also be prescribed by homeopaths, and salts for asthmatic conditions are mag phos, kali phos, kali mur and nat mur. Homeopathic remedies are available from some pharmacies, and from practitioners.

Homeopathy was popular in the nineteenth century, but as orthodox medicine began to have great success treating dangerous diseases with a new generation of drugs – the antibiotics and their relatives – support for homeopathy waned. Several research studies have shown the effectiveness of homeopathy. In the U.S. homeopathic remedies are regulated by the FDA as over-the-counter drugs. Homeopathy was the medicine of the past and its adherents believe it will become the medicine of the future. The ever-increasing sales of homeopathic remedies are evidence that its popularity is growing strongly.

Biochemical Tissue Salts

In the late 1800s William Schuessler, a German physician, originated what he called a biochemic system of medicine. He identified 12 "tissue salts" which he claimed were vital for health and could cure simple, everyday ailments. Schuessler believed that not only was disease an unnatural condition and at variance with the intentions of nature, but that within the body itself were the most potent weapons in the battle against disease. Healing could be stimulated by natural, recuperative forces within the body. The way to stimulate the body was through redressing imbalances in the system by taking his tissue salts.

Dr. Schuessler developed these mineral salts in an easily assimilated form. The amount of minerals in the tissue salts is in fact tiny, much smaller than would generally be given as a supplement, but the purpose of them is not to make up for dietary deficiencies but to arouse the body to heal itself. They are therefore a kind of homeopathic remedy, and are prescribed on the same principles.

The Schuessler minerals most commonly used in the treatment of asthma are potassium phosphate (kali phos), potassium chloride (kali mur), magnesium phosphate (mag phos) and sodium chloride (nat mur). Which remedy is selected depends on the particular condition, for instance whether it is bronchial asthma, nervous asthma, if it is accompanied by fever, is worse in the evening or in an overheated room.

The relevant symptoms are best assessed by an experienced practitioner. It is advisable, therefore, that you consult a naturopath or homeopath for a proper diagnosis. Tissue salts at low potencies are available from reputable health food stores but higher potencies can be obtained from practitioners. As the tablets are generally lactose-based anyone with a milk-sugar intolerance should be wary of taking regular preparations.

Tissue salts are said to relieve short-term conditions such as colds and flu quickly but long-standing ailments and chronic conditions such as asthma could take six months or more to respond. Tissue salts and homeopathic remedies do not conflict with other forms of treatment or prescribed medication but serious conditions should always be treated under medical supervision. Taking them does not mean you should stop any pharmaceutical medication for asthma, but it may be possible to reduce your need for it.

Bach Flower Remedies

As recently as 1930 Edward Bach, a British medical doctor and bacteriologist, developed a system of remedies designed to treat the whole person, not just symptoms of illness.

Dr. Bach believed that the basis of disease was the disharmony between the spiritual and mental aspects of human nature. He developed his remedies from well-known flowers and plants. The principle behind their use is that every disorder – physical or psychological – arises because of an inner imbalance for which nature has provided a cure, in the form of healing plants, sunlight, spring water and fresh air.

It is certainly true that asthma can be the result of mental disharmony and imbalance: stress is known to cause asthma, and fear is a potent trigger. Additionally the body's vitality may be lowered as a result of asthma, which in turn can result in unhappiness, depression, feelings of inadequacy, and so on.

The flower remedies of Dr. Bach are selected according to the mental and emotional state of the patient and not on any physical disorder. As the mind is both delicate and sensitive, the remedies need to be selected with great care. Where asthmatics suffer anguish, sweet chestnut would be the remedy. If they lack confidence, cerato would be prescribed. If there is drowsiness, then clematis could help, or if they suffer exhaustion through strain and effort, then vervain might be suggested.

Many people carry with them a small bottle of a combination of Bach flowers called Rescue Remedy. It is a mixture of star of Bethlehem, rock rose, impatiens, cherry plum and clematis. This is especially helpful in emergency situations, for example an acute attack of asthma, times of sudden shock, fright or emotional trauma. It is said by supporters of the system that Bach flowers should be the first thing to use in an emergency and the last thing to use when all else has failed.

Many people have testified to the effectiveness of Dr. Bach's series of preparations. Diane, a patient in her fifties, experienced crippling asthma attacks. Not only did she suffer chronic asthma but also extreme anxiety, nervousness, depression and fear. This was caused by her husband, who came home intoxicated most nights and would fly into fits of rage. This behavior had continued for years. Bach flower preparations of olive, gorse, centuary and agrimony were chosen to allay her fear and anxiety. After a period of time, Diane became more assertive and sought counseling, gaining support to help her cope with her difficulties. Diane now suffers fewer asthma attacks, feels stronger in herself and more capable of coping with her husband.

A second example is that of Michelle, a sixteen-year-old girl, who had the very common symptoms of extreme tiredness, irritability, premenstrual tension, constipation and asthma with severe wheezing. As well as taking her puffer medication, Michelle was encouraged to take selected Bach flower remedies and spend some time on Controlled Pattern Breathing and relaxation techniques. The mustard, olive, larch and impatiens remedies were chosen for her. Michelle is now an entirely different girl and basically free of her symptoms.

Bach flower remedies have no side effects and can be used in conjunction with orthodox treatment. They are safe for babies and children. They are freely available in pharmacies, health food stores and natural therapy stores. Dr. Bach intended his remedies to be simple enough for anyone to use without consulting a professional but if you are in doubt about what category your emotional state could be described as, you can consult a trained practitioner or Bach therapist for an individual prescription. Dr. Bach taught that not more than five preparations should be used at one time. They are taken by placing drops under the tongue night and morning.

The Bach Society gives the following guidelines for the remedies and the type of personality they are intended to treat.

AGRIMONY	*Those who hide worries behind a cheerful face.*
ASPEN	*Apprehensive for no known reason.*
BEECH	*Those critical and intolerant of others.*
CENTUARY	*Weak-willed, easily exploited or imposed upon.*
CERATO	*Those who doubt their own judgement, seek confirmation from others.*
CHERRY PLUM	*Those suffering from tension, fear, uncontrolled or irrational thoughts.*
CHESTNUT BUD	*Refuses to learn by experience and continually repeats same mistakes.*
CHICORY	*Possessive (self-centered), clinging and overprotective, especially to loved ones.*
CLEMATIS	*Inattentive, dreamy, absent-minded, escapist.*
CRAB APPLE	*The "cleanser" for self disgust, prudishness, shame at ailments.*
ELM	*Feelings of inadequacy, overwhelming responsibility.*
GENTIAN	*Despondency.*
GORSE	*Feelings of hopelessness, pessimism, defeatism.*
HEATHER	*Talkative (obsessed with own troubles and experiences).*
HOLLY	*Hatred, envy, jealousy, suspicion.*
HONEYSUCKLE	*Living in the past, nostalgia, homesickness.*
HORNBEAM	*"Monday morning" feeling, mental fatigue, procrastination.*
IMPATIENS	*Impatience, irritability.*
LARCH	*Lack of self-confidence, feelings of inferiority, fear of failure.*
MIMULUS	*Fear of known things, shyness, timidity.*
MUSTARD	*"Dark cloud" that descends, feeling sad and low for no reason.*
OAK	*Naturally strong/courageous, but no longer able to struggle bravely against illness or adversity.*
OLIVE	*Exhaustion, feeling drained of energy by long-standing problems.*
PINE	*Guilt, blaming oneself even for the mistakes of others. Always apologizing.*

RED CHESTNUT	*Obsessed by care and concern for others.*
ROCK ROSE	*Suddenly alarmed, scared, panicky.*
ROCK WATER	*Rigid minded, self-denying.*
SCLERANTHUS	*For those with uncertainty/indecision/ vacillation; fluctuating moods.*
STAR OF BETHLEHEM	*For all the effects of serious news, or fright, following an accident, shock and grief.*
SWEET CHESTNUT	*Utter dejection, bleak outlook, despair.*
VERVAIN	*For those with overenthusiasm, fanatical beliefs.*
VINE	*Dominating, inflexible, tyrannical, autocratic, arrogant. Usually good leaders.*
WALNUT	*Assists in adjustment to transition or change, e.g. puberty, menopause, divorce, new surroundings.*
WATER VIOLET	*Proud, reserved, aloof; enjoys being alone.*
WHITE CHESTNUT	*Persistent unwanted thoughts. Preoccupation with some worry or episode. Mental conflict.*
WILD OAT	*Unsure of direction in life.*
WILD ROSE	*Resignation, apathy.*
WILLOW	*For those who are resentful, embittered, always thinking "poor old me."*

Californian flower essences

Using the principles of the Bach flower remedies, other countries discovered and developed remedies using their own plants, flowers and trees. Thus North America has the Californian flower essences and Australia the bush flower essences. These once local essences are now being distributed all over the world.

Readily available throughout the U.S., the range of Californian flower remedies is so extensive that only a few can be mentioned here. The following are included because of their particular relevance to helping asthma.

CHAMOMILE	*Helps soothe nervousness, due to anxiety and anger, creating calm and harmony.*

DILL ESSENCE	*For jaded nerves caused by a too-busy lifestyle.*
NASTURTIUM	*To regain mental and physical vitality.*
PENSTEMON	*Provides courage and confidence to persevere, changes a pessimistic attitude to optimistic.*
PINK YARROW	*For strengthening the body's vitality and counteracting the effects of negative emotions.*
SCARLET MONKEYFLOWER	*Helps release pent-up anger, resentment, fear and emotional stress.*
SCOTCH BROOM	*Used when lack of motivation, doubt and discouragement causes an imbalance in the body to the point of depression.*
YARROW	*For those who have become drained by city life and its stresses.*

Australian bush flower essences

The Australian Aborigines have always used flowers to heal emotional imbalances and physical injuries, and so it is no surprise that Australian native flowers have proved to be suitable for making remedies in the tradition of Bach flowers.

Australian plants have a real beauty and strength, and since Australia is relatively unpolluted and metaphysically has a very wise old energy, the plants are considered to carry the inherent power of the land. This makes the Australian bush flower remedies quite unique.

The bush flower remedies are intended to give clarity to one's life and the courage, strength and enthusiasm to pursue goals and dreams. They are said to assist self esteem, enhance intuition and creativity, increase vitality and energy, help emotional balance, release negative beliefs and thoughts and enhance survival skills in crises. All these are ideal attitudes for someone with asthma to develop, so they can confidently and positively take control of their condition.

Although 50 preparations are available, below are listed just a few particularly recommended to create harmony, better health and well-being for asthmatics.

BAUHINIA	*For those resistant to change, rigid, annoyed. Will result in embracing new concepts and ideas; acceptance and open-mindedness.*
BLACK-EYED SUSAN	*For the stressed, rushing, constantly striving, impatient. Results in slowing down, ability to be still, inner peace.*
CROWEA	*For worry, sense of feeling "not quite right." Results in balancing and centering the individual, vitality.*
DOG ROSE	*For the shy, insecure; apprehensive. Results in confidence, courage, belief in self.*
FIVE CORNERS	*For low self-esteem, dislike of self, "held-in" personality. Results in love and acceptance of self.*
GREY SPIDER FLOWER	*Terror, panic. Results in faith, courage.*
ILLAWARRA FLAME TREE	*Sense of rejection, feeling of being left out, fear of responsibility. Results in self approval, self reliance, confidence, inner strength.*
MACROCARPA	*Tired, burnt out, low immunity. Remedy has strong affinity to the adrenal glands, bringing energy, strength and vitality.*
OLD MAN BANKSIA	*Lethargy, low in energy, sluggish, disheartened, weary, those with low thyroid activity. Regains energy, enthusiasm and interest in life.*
PEACH FLOWERED TEA-TREE	*Mood swings, lack of commitment, hypochondriacs. Results in emotional balance, completion of goals and projects, trust and responsibility in own health.*
WARATAH	*Despair, hopelessness, inability to respond to crisis. Results in courage, tenacity, strong faith, adaptability, survival skills.*
WILD POTATO BUSH	*Sense of being physically encumbered and weighed down – body not able to respond as one would wish. Outcome is vitality.*

Aromatherapy

The principles of aromatherapy are ancient although the term itself is new. Egyptian priests of Cleopatra's time used aromatic oils to help heal the sick, but it was French chemist Rene-Maurice Gattefosse, early in the twentieth century, who coined the word **aromatherapie**. Apparently he discovered that the many oils used in perfumes were better antiseptics and healing substances than the formulas available at the time. Gattefosse found out the hard way: he burnt his hand one day and plunged it into a bowl of lavender oil, mistaking it for water. The burn healed quickly and without a scar.

Aromatherapy makes therapeutic use of essential oils extracted from nature's kingdom: from flowers, trees, bushes, roots, seeds, herbs and even bark. Essential oils are the substances which give plants their aromas; however, the aroma is only one aspect of their total constituents and properties. Often referred to as the soul of the plant, they are a combination of a large number of compounds which together produce powerful therapeutic effects. When essential oils are extracted from plants these healing properties are harvested. These valuable essences contain vitamins, hormones and cell regenerating agents, to nourish, energize and protect. They are believed to work in two ways: directly on the body and on the emotions.

Aromatherapy is currently enjoying renewed popularity due to the availability of an extensive variety of oils, the ease with which they can be incorporated into our lives, and the range of emotional changes they can produce in us. They can be used to invigorate our senses when we wake or soothe and calm us at the close of a busy day.

Well-known British aromatherapist Shirley Price believes aromatherapy helps bring feelings of anger, jealousy, fear and resentment to the surface – stopping them from turning into physical health problems. She advocates the daily use of oils for skin, body and general health care, to strengthen the immune system by keeping infections at bay. She points out that the principal organs of detoxification in the body – the skin, lungs, intestines, liver, kidneys and lymph glands – benefit from the cleansing and energizing properties of many oils.

Whether or not we are aware of it, the smells that surround

us daily can change our mood by either lifting or lowering our spirits. Many essential oils are linked to our emotions, to improve harmony and balance in our lives. They have a significant effect on our moods and energy levels. They can be uplifting, calming, invigorating – or simply have an appeal to our sense of smell, which passes reactive messages to our brain.

Modern medical circles are beginning to recognize the merits of aromatherapy. Therapists are now visiting hospitals, nursing homes and hospices with their fragrant essences, practicing aromatherapy in tandem with naturopathy, remedial massage and beauty therapy.

Robert Tisserand, in his book *Aromatherapy for Everyone* (Penguin), divides aromatherapy into three main areas: clinical, holistic and aesthetic. In clinical or medical aromatherapy, essential oils are prescribed along with herbal preparations to treat disease. This is especially popular with doctors in France. Holistic aromatherapy combines oils and massage to treat a range of health problems of the mind, body and spirit. The holistic approach also takes into account nutrition, subtle energy imbalances, counseling and skin care. Esthetic aromatherapy is the use of oils by beauty therapists to treat skin problems and aid relaxation and weight control.

Stress is a huge emotional burden, so it is no surprise to find that many common stress-based disorders such as PMS, eczema, acne, psoriasis, chronic fatigue syndrome, digestive disturbances, insomnia, sinusitis, headaches, muscular aches and pains respond well to aromatherapy. Stress is also a trigger for asthma, so aromatherapy can play a part in its treatment too.

The antifungal and antibacterial properties of essential oils also supply the asthmatic with protection against airborne viruses and bacteria. Their aromatic vapors silently penetrate blocked airways, to keep them clear and make breathing easier. At their simplest, refreshing and aromatic essential oils will keep your home fragrant and fresh by removing stale and unwanted odors. You can use just one aromatic oil or a blend of many oils.

What particular smells do you like or dislike? Think about it! Perhaps there are a few – or many – which have an adverse effect on you. Then there are the wonderful smells that simply make you feel good. What are they? Make a list and with very little effort you can create your own pleasurable, aromatic environment. Just imagine the therapeutic boost you can give yourself with essential oils.

Marjoram, Roman chamomile, myrrh, lavender, juniper, wintergreen and tea tree are recognized as the most beneficial essential oils for people with asthma, along with the indispensable eucalyptus. Chamomile calms inflammation and allergies. Myrrh is known to be an expectorant and has anti-inflammatory properties. Marjoram, a sedating oil, is calming to the emotions and will promote a deep and restful sleep. Lavender balances the thyroid gland and small intestine, and releases acute nervous exhaustion, depression and frustration. Juniper balances the thyroid and the bladder and releases acute anxiety and stress from no known cause. Tea tree is excellent for all types of infection, an aid to strengthening the immune system and helping to fight invading organisms. There is also evidence that tea tree oil helps control dust mites. Eucalyptus will relieve the discomfort of congested nasal passages, open up the airways and help stop the spread of infection. It is such an excellent remedy for asthma that more information is given about it later (see overleaf).

Essential oils are quickly absorbed into the skin via the hair follicles so massage is the most effective way to experience the benefits of aromatherapy. Full of vitality and natural energy, essential oils will rejuvenate and stimulate the skin's natural functions. Two or three drops of eucalyptus, lavender, marjoram and juniper oils together, in 25 ml of a carrier oil, is adequate for a relaxing full body massage. Suitable carrier oils are apricot, sweet almond, avocado, jojoba, grapeseed, olive, wheat germ and safflower. Essential oils should almost always be diluted; lavender, a good all-rounder which can enliven or relax, is the only oil that can be used neat – but then only on adults.

Other effective ways to use essential oils are to add 2–3 drops to an oil burner, for a fragrant home or work place; or add a few drops to your bathwater for a blissful experience. A few drops of oil in a bowl of steaming water will create healing aromatic vapors to clear away congestion and restore comfort to your body. A drop of chamomile, marjoram or lavender oil on your pillowcase will lull you off to sleep. There is nothing new about perfumed bed linen for in the Middle Ages laundresses would drape the household sheets over lavender bushes to dry and impart the plant's fresh, clean scent.

Although strong-smelling substances, fragrances and perfumes can actually provoke asthma attacks in some people, pure essential oils contain no irritating additives to aggravate. Nevertheless, someone with asthma who is unsure of possible adverse reactions should start by using essential oils sparingly.

EUCALYPTUS

A great deal of Australian history can be traced from the bushmen who first distilled eucalyptus from the leaves of the blue mallee gum tree, in the very early days of settlement in Australia. Although almost all Australian gum trees are eucalypts, this particular species contains the most aromatic and potent oil, and so is the most suitable to harvest from. Today, the blue mallee gum grows in abundance throughout the world, so the oil is also produced worldwide.

Eucalyptus oil is probably the most effective and natural remedy to help reduce the severity of an asthma attack. It can also prevent attacks even starting, as the vapor stops airways becoming dry and so reduces upper respiratory tract infections. There are specific vaporizers on the market, to help relieve asthma, croup, head colds and respiratory ailments, and you can add eucalyptus oil to make the vapor more effective. Eucalyptus massaged into the chest before bed will help those who tend to wake during the night with asthma.

When early warnings of asthma such as mild wheezing appear, place one or two drops of eucalyptus oil in a bowl with steaming hot water, drape a towel over your head and inhale the vapor. This will also help to clear the head and ease nasal congestion if you have a cold or influenza. Likewise, a few drops on a handkerchief can be inhaled throughout the day to keep your nasal passages clear. Sprinkle one or two drops on your pillow for a pleasant night's sleep.

The therapeutic properties of eucalyptus go beyond asthma and respiratory problems, though, as it is also an effective remedy for muscular aches and pains, and insect bites. Eucalyptus can be used as a mouthwash and bath refresher, as a hand and skin cleanser or in a vaporizer, humidifier and in a sauna. Eucalyptus nasal sprays, joint and muscle ointments and chest rubs are available – even eucalyptus sweets with lemon and honey.

Eucalyptus is an effective antiseptic so can be used (diluted) on wounds. Try it for headaches by rubbing one or two drops gently around your temple area. It has been used as a scalp massage to help control dandruff. Add one or two drops to a small quantity of carrier oil and use for a complete body massage (but not for babies). A few drops in your bathwater will create a soothing and relaxing effect – and remember that relaxation is an important factor in the management of asthma.

Eucalyptus will protect your whole environment. Use it as your disinfectant, room deodorizer, insect repellent and spot cleaner. A limited amount in the dishwasher and washing machine will disinfect your dishes and clothes. Place one or two drops in the dog's bath water to rid him of fleas and make him smell nice. Don't forget to use one or two drops in the car to eliminate unwanted fumes and for a refreshing drive to work!

For a more efficient distribution of the aroma you can use a fan-forced, air-filtered vaporizer and add the oil to it. This safe, slow-release system can be used in rooms with limited ventilation to help relieve asthma and respiratory conditions. A smaller version of this air vaporizer has been designed to sit snugly on the air vents of cars.

Discovering the many and varied uses of all essential oils, not just eucalyptus, will take you on a delightful aromatic journey to uplift your spirit and enliven you physically and emotionally. Enjoy these wonderful feelings of discovery and revel in the use of essential oils. Take time to pamper yourself – you deserve it. Relax, enjoy life and watch your health and your asthma improve.

HANDS-ON THERAPIES

Chiropractic

The doctor of the future shall provide no drugs but interest his patients in the care of the spine.

Thomas Edison (1847–1933)

The word chiropractic is derived from the Greek words **cheiro**, meaning hand, and **practikos**, practical, and describes the modality: it is done by hand. Chiropractic is a method of healing human diseases and injuries by adjusting the body. It has increased in popularity in more recent years, and in most countries it is now fully accepted as a natural and effective healing method.

Daniel David Palmer, a Canadian who worked in the latter half of the last century, is recognized as the founder of modern chiropractic, but less scientific methods were being applied in various cultures long before Palmer's time. Witch doctors in Africa often performed cures, even "miracles," by walking on someone's back, up and down the spine. The ancient Chinese, Egyptians, Brazilians and people in Southeast Asian countries also practiced a type of chiropractic adjustment.

Today we are more scientific. Chiropractic is not a healing approach that aims to be a cure-all, but instead it tries to rectify muscular and skeletal disorders and so energize the nervous system and activate the body to heal itself. The premise of chiropractic is related to Newton's Third Law of Motion, that to every action there is an equal and opposite reaction. Chiropractic asserts that the nervous system controls all other systems in the body and interference with the nerves will impair the functioning of the body. This may lead to disease, by making the body less resistant to infection.

An analogy might be that when a tree is ringbarked it dies because the natural energies previously flowing through the trunk and up to the leaves have been restricted, so the leaves slowly wither and die. Likewise if there is a nerve root impingement coming from the spinal cord or its extending nerves, then there will be reduction in overall energy flow, generally to the peripheral areas of the body. Over time the body, like the ringbarked tree, is likely to suffer: colds, flu, headaches or other relatively mild complaints. Unless the body's energy flow is restored, the problems will gradually worsen and become chronic.

The human spinal column is long, and is prone to misalignment and minor dislocation – as the result of accident, hereditary defects or generally poor posture over a long period. Throughout life, people constantly suffer minor injuries like a fall, sudden shock, a sporting injury, muscle tissue damage, whiplash from an automobile accident. As a result the spine's alignment may be altered and may **remain** out of alignment, causing a "nerve root impingement." Symptoms may include tingling in the arms, cold fingers or hands, pains in the lower back or legs, upper arm aches, tennis elbow, more frequent colds and sore throats than usual, tightness in the chest, shortness of breath, wheezing, stiff neck, headache, sinus problems – and asthma. No particular significance may be attached to the injury at the time. The onset of the resultant symptoms may be gradual, not becoming apparent until six months or more after the injury.

Chiropractors are trained to make a diagnosis and then to adjust the spine to correct the misalignment which may be causing the problem. Before making any adjustment tests are carried out to identify the faulty alignment and any existing neurological problems. Analyses may be made using X-rays and other imaging machines, and nerve impulses may be measured.

Tests and treatments are carried out on a couch, which can be raised or lowered by the chiropractor. Adjustments are usually made manually; however, sometimes firm, wedge-shaped 'blocks' are placed around the back or pelvic area to re-align the spine. A high-pressure activator is often used to apply pressure quickly and firmly and some chiropractic adjustments can be more effective with a "dropped table" technique. Parts of a spring-loaded, recoil-action couch or table can drop about 5 mm, in line with the part of the body being treated, and this accentuates the movement required for the adjustment.

Chiropractic care may sound rough but is in fact very gentle and does not cause any undue discomfort. In most cases very little movement or pressure is applied to the various parts of the body or spinal column. Sometimes when an adjustment is made close to the patient's ears a cracking noise can be heard. This is simply the joint moving as pressure on the nerve is relieved.

There are a number of chiropractic methods – Logan, Stillwell, Thompson and Diversified being some. However, the basic objective is the same for all: to relieve nerve root impingement, restore normal nerve transmission and promote a return to good health. Chiropractic is not limited to treating any one disease because it searches for, and endeavors to remove, the causes of ill health rather than treating the symptoms.

Chiropractic has no age barriers. Babies born with the use of forceps often sustain neck or spine strain that can be treated. Adolescents' growing pains can be the result of musculoskeletal injury from seemingly minor falls or accidents when they were younger. Senior citizens' back or joint pain can often be helped.

Chiropractic now enjoys worldwide acceptance. It is no longer considered "alternative," and a growing number of health insurance plans around the world cover chiropractic in the same way as orthodox medical consultations. The chiropractor works in a close relationship with other health practitioners.

ASTHMA AND CHIROPRACTIC
Asthma is believed by chiropractors to be mainly related to the position of the first and second thoracic vertebrae (the ones at the top of your back), although misalignment of the spine in

other areas can be a contributing factor. Faulty alignment around the seventh cervical vertebra (at the base of the neck) can also be a reason for asthma and breathing difficulties.

Spine.

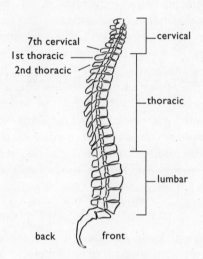

7th cervical
1st thoracic
2nd thoracic

cervical

thoracic

lumbar

back   front

Osteopathy

Dr. Andrew Taylor Still worked in Missouri in the nineteenth century. He founded osteopathy after he became discontented with orthodox medicine – three of his children caught viral meningitis and he was unable to save them using his medical skills and the drugs then available.

Before turning to medicine he had studied engineering and this, along with his knowledge of anatomy, made him look on the body as a machine. He theorized that many illnesses were the result of the framework of bones, joints, muscles and ligaments being out of alignment. Disease was the result of interference to the blood supply or nerves, caused by abnormalities in or near joints or vertebrae, and manipulation would restore balance and cure the illness. Releasing nerves and blood supply in particular parts of the body would, he taught, set up a reaction with the hormone system and thus mobilize the healing process.

Osteopathy is today one of the most widely used complementary forms of medicine. It is especially popular in the United
States, where most of the modern research done on its effects
has been conducted. The osteopath aims to restore the harmony
and structural integrity of the body. The technique consists primarily of adjustments (slight movement of vertebrae or bone) to
the spine and other bones and joints.

Osteopathy is not, however, limited to adjustments in the
way chiropractic is. A practitioner may also correct posture with
simple exercises and toning of body muscles. Other treatments
are also important: to ensure the lymphatic and blood systems'
drainage is working efficiently and to improve arterial blood
flow. Treatments used in conjunction with osteopathy may
include immunology, prescription medicine, psychology and
other modern disciplines. The osteopath will often use electrical
or mechanical equipment, heat, massage, hydrotherapy or recommend surgery if necessary.

Chiropractors and osteopaths do, however, share a similar
philosophy. Many colleges have faculties in both chiropractic
and osteopathy with undergraduate studies running side by side.
In some countries many medical practitioners are also osteopaths.

OSTEOPATHY AND ASTHMA

Osteopathic techniques may improve asthma as they invigorate
the blood and nerve supplies. Consequently the patient's general
health improves, which in turn improves the asthmatic condition.
Although osteopaths also believe that good health depends upon
good nutrition, a clean environment and other conditions associated with a healthy way of life – all of which improve
asthma – their main emphasis is on the muscular-skeletal system
and the interrelationship of this with other parts of the body.

Kinesiology

Kinesiology, derived from the Greek word **kinesis** meaning
"motion," is the science of purposeful muscle movement in the
body. Adherents believe that muscle testing can detect various
imbalances in the body, which can then be corrected. Kinesiologists do not claim to diagnose illnesses, but teach that the

response of the muscles is a guide to pinpointing all kinds of physical problems.

G. Goodheart, an American doctor of chiropractic, is recognized as the originator of applied kinesiology. He determined that when the muscles are in good working order, so is the body, and his research further discovered that each muscle group related to particular parts of the body – the heart, lungs, digestive system, glands, bones, circulation and so on.

Muscles are reliant on good supplies of blood and lymph – the body fluid which drains the tissues via the lymphatic system, carrying away toxins and substances to be excreted – to keep healthy. Kinesiologists try to enhance the blood flow to the muscles and balance the lymphatic system by stimulating appropriate pressure points. In addition, kinesiologists believe that an invisible energy controls our bodily functions, much like a computer circuit controls a washing-machine cycle. These circuits can "blow a fuse" during illness or if we are under stress, devitalizing our body. The practitioner can check these by muscle testing and then reset out-of-balance circuits.

Gentle manual pressure tests the muscle response and reveals to the practitioner how a specific area is functioning. A weakened muscle can indicate an energy level problem in its associated organ. A light fingertip massage on pressure points of the body and scalp will revitalize any pinpointed trouble spots.

Kinesiologists believe that allergic reactions to nutrients and chemicals affect, among other things, the way our muscles work and their response to testing. Various allergies respond extremely well to applied kinesiology (and asthma has an allergic basis in many cases), but you should take into account that the kinesiologist may be recommending changes in lifestyle, such as reducing stress, improving your diet or taking supplements, that will also be having an effect on the allergy.

The muscle testing is painless. A simple test involves having a patient extend an arm horizontally and, on demand, tightening and holding the arm firm while the practitioner applies downward pressure. The ability of the patient to exert an equal and opposite pressure is assessed by the practitioner, and if the muscle does not respond normally a series of touch tests are made to find out why.

A similar approach has been developed by Dr. John

Diamond, with refinements. His technique is called behavioral kinesiology, and integrates psychiatry and psychosomatic medicine with kinesiology. Dr. Diamond explained his philosophy in a book *Your Body Does Not Lie* (Warner Books, New York): "I would practice preventative medicine, which meant raising the patient's energy to overcome the earliest manifestations of disease or better to act to prevent disease from occurring in the first place." Such an approach is common to many workers in the field of complementary medicine.

Behavioral kinesiology is not unlike applied physiology, a powerful system of stress management procedures developed by an American, Richard Utt. Using deep, accurate muscle testing procedures and monitoring techniques, applied physiology evaluates stress in various parts of the nervous system.

Although broad muscle testing procedures and techniques are specific to trained practitioners, kinesiology is practiced by many people, including chiropractors, osteopaths and natural therapists worldwide.

KINESIOLOGY AND ASTHMA
Kinesiology may be able to identify an asthmatic condition when the response from testing specific muscles relating to the lung is weak. The diaphragm spindle cells (nerve cells in the muscle) are considered to be particularly important in relation to breathing difficulties and fatigue.

Touch for health

Touch for health is a modified form of kinesiology which uses a series of muscle tests to identify physical imbalances and emotional disharmony. The founder, Dr. John Thie, an American chiropractor, claims it can help relieve aches and pains, improve posture, eliminate tension, enliven energy levels, help to prevent illness, promote relaxation and well-being. Fault corrections are made using massage or light touch techniques which it is said will restore the body's flow of energy. Essentially this is a discipline that lay people learn and practice, rather than professionals, and classes are held regularly in most countries.

Massage

Massage is something most of us naturally do almost every day. When we suffer an injury, stiffness or an ache, we instinctively rub or apply pressure to the part of the body that hurts.

Probably the oldest form of medical treatment, massage was used by ancient Chinese, Indian and Egyptian cultures to prevent and cure diseases and heal injuries. The ancient Greeks and Romans advocated massage before and after sport, instead of exercise during recuperation from illness, or as a medical treatment for such diverse conditions as melancholia, asthma, digestive problems and even sterility. The Greek father of medicine, Hippocrates, wrote in the fifth century BC, "The way to health is to have a scented bath and an oiled massage each day." Indians have always valued massage and Ayurvedic treatments – a system of medicine dating back to 1800 BC – use massage to rub remedial herbs, spices and aromatic oils into the skin.

Massage grew in popularity in the Western world from the nineteenth century, influenced by Per Henrik Ling (1776–1839), a Swedish gymnast. His treatments are what is known today as Swedish massage. Apart from traditional Swedish massage there is a variety of massage practices, which focus on healing as well as creating and maintaining good health. In the 1970s, George Downing, an American massage therapist, published a trend-setting work entitled *The Massage Book* in which he formulated the idea of massage as a therapy to relax, stimulate and invigorate mind and body.

Massage systems available in the Western world are aimed at being remedial, structural or functional. They include such therapies as deep tissue massage, the Bowen technique, mobilization massage, movement integration, and therapeutic or relaxation massage. Eastern massage systems such as shiatsu are also widely practiced, as is acupressure, a massage-like refinement using the theory of acupuncture points.

The main massage movements are:

- **effleurage** – light, slow, rhythmic, surface stroking usually with the palms and fingertips
- **petrissage** – medium pressure kneading, squeezing, rolling and releasing to warm the muscles

- **friction** – heavy, small, circular movements made with
  one or more fingers, the heel of the hand or pads of
  the thumbs to relieve muscle tension
- **percussion or tapotement** – short, fast, rhythmic,
  drumming movements using the cupped palms of the
  hands, delivered briskly but lightly
- **vibration** – trembling movement
- **rolfing** – heavy pressure (see pages 147–8).

A relaxation massage uses only the first three or four movements,
finishing off with effleurage or light stroking, and is one of life's
great delights. Psychologically and emotionally its calming and
soothing effects ease anxiety, stress, tension and depression and
simply make you feel good.

Physically, massage improves the blood, muscular and
nervous systems and helps the body assimilate food and eliminate
waste. Massage can be used to treat circulation problems and
help high blood pressure, headaches, hyperactivity, insomnia,
sinusitis and breathing problems. Nurses and physiotherapists
massage patients to promote circulation to the muscles of bed-
ridden patients and to help relieve pain or physical discomfort.
Deep and intense pressure massage eases the stiffness often experienced by athletes and dancers, by draining waste products
which accumulate in muscles after strenuous activity.

Massage is not suitable for people with a fever, blood
poisoning, hemorrhaging, vein inflammation or varicose veins,
thrombosis, spinal disease, acute inflammation, tumors, skin
disease, pregnancy, abscesses, tubercular joints, severe abdominal
pain, a heart condition or in the throes of an asthma attack.

A full body massage should take about 50–60 minutes, while
just the back and upper body would only take 30–45 minutes,
but massage to a localised area may be for only 5–15 minutes.

Masseurs apply different techniques and approaches depending on their particular training. It is important you seek a qualified and reputable masseur.

Without a doubt, a weekly massage will improve your
overall well-being, whether it is for a medical condition or just
to relieve stress. If you are in any doubt, try it for three months
and experience the luxury of being pampered – a glorious feeling
that modern drugs cannot match.

MASSAGE AND ASTHMA

When an asthma sufferer is feeling well, a face, head and neck massage will stimulate the circulation through the tissues of the face and impede mucus build-up in the sinuses. An upper body massage can move mucus lower down, in the bronchial passages.

Lying on a massage couch can inhibit the breathing of some people with asthma, but they can still be massaged when sitting on a chair. Most professional masseurs now have ergonomically designed massage chairs particularly for this purpose. Having the shoulders, scapula and each side of the spinal column massaged is especially appropriate for asthmatics and can be comfortably carried out in a seated position.

Rolfing

Rolfing is not suitable for children.

Rolfing is a complex manipulative system initiated early in the 1930s by Dr. Ida Rolf, designed to correct poor body posture. Dr. Rolf believed that abnormal posture put such a strain on the body that it drained it of vitality and left it open to illness. She taught that realigning the body into a straight vertical line would restore the body to normal working order.

Rolfing uses extreme pressure and deep massage, often using the elbows to penetrate deeply into muscle tissue – which can be quite painful. This loosens connective tissue and muscles, which encourages the fibers to return to their correct position.

Rolfing has gained acceptance as an effective deep-penetrating massage technique which requires less energy to be expended by the masseur than other massage systems. It enables a person of limited stature to apply deep pressure over the area to be penetrated, by using their full body weight.

ROLFING AND ASTHMA

Rolfing can be very effective in correcting the hunched posture assumed by some asthmatics, and for loosening and breaking up muscle tension around the spinal column and scapular region. Pain tolerance levels must be considered and need to be carefully monitored but, provided the patient can cope with this treatment, rolfing is suitable for adults who believe the cause of their distress is due to a misaligned body structure.

Mobilization Massage

Mobilization massage is not suitable for children.

Mobilization massage is a specific technique studied by clinical masseurs who undertake postgraduate courses. It is used to help asthma, chest and diaphragm. Primarily designed to increase the diaphragm's ability to inhale and exhale air, mobilization massage relaxes the muscles in and around the rib cage and sternum to make breathing easier. This results in increased air intake.

Mobilization massage can be rather uncomfortable as it involves rib and intercostal (between the ribs) muscle release, so before a session the patient is given a general massage for complete relaxation and to nurture confidence in the skills of the practitioner. The actual procedure involves "pumping" the ribs and sternum (the breastbone) where they meet by pushing on them alternately, and also producing a shearing action across the ribs. This deep pressure work can be quite painful. The technique is so specific that it requires expertise in assessing and using pressure to just below the pain threshold of the particular patient.

Patients feel noticeably different after just one treatment. Each session takes about an hour and several sessions are usually needed to gain benefit from this method. Patients also need to learn the importance of correct postural habits and how to adjust their individual body movements.

There are many practitioners of mobilization massage in the U.S. and the U.K. In Australia a related form of the massage, respiratory mobilization, is gaining ground.

MOBILIZATION MASSAGE AND ASTHMA

Mobilization massage has been shown to increase the lung and diaphragm function of asthma sufferers, but not everyone can endure the discomfort associated with the shearing action.

Bowen Technique

Tom Bowen was born in Geelong, Victoria, Australia and died in 1982. Bowen had little medical training, but like many other people, had discovered the strength of the healing relationship between mind and body. He believed that our unique energy systems can be affected by our emotions, nutrition and environment – the same critical factors which affect so many people with asthma.

Bowen was able to detect minute changes in muscle tension and so developed a dynamic system of muscle and connective tissue moves to balance the body and stimulate energy flow. Bowen treated thousands of people every year with his gentle, negative and positive moves, and was known to restore people to good health with only two treatments seven days apart. In recent years followers have established Bowen Therapy academies and there are now many practitioners over the world, especially in Canada, the U.S. and New Zealand.

Bowen technique pressure is light but firm. The therapist uses two or four fingers to gently roll muscles from side to side. Known as the **golgi tendon reflex**, this triggers muscles to relax and penetrates deeply to rebalance energy levels, correct skeletal irregularities and improve body posture.

BOWEN TECHNIQUE AND ASTHMA

Many asthma sufferers have reported that the Bowen technique has given them a new lease on life. Long-standing conditions have been eliminated, the discomfort of their asthma has been eased and their mobility has been restored.

Muscles around the rib cage, under the sternum, under the diaphragm, either side of the spine from base to neck, and in the upper back are most usually focused on to help asthma.

Reflexology

Some 85 years ago, William H. Fitzgerald, M.D., created an interest in an ancient Chinese and Indian pressure therapy in which soles of the feet and, less commonly, palms of the hands, are massaged to prompt the body to heal itself. This "zone therapy," as it was called by the Chinese around 3000 BC and then by

William Fitzgerald, was further developed around 1920 by Edwin Bowers, M.D., and in the 1930s by Eunice Ingham, who concentrated solely on the feet.

Today, trained reflexologists worldwide are successfully treating and preventing diseases in various parts of the body by massaging relevant "reflex areas" in the feet. Numerous books have now been written on the subject and reflexologists believe that good results have been achieved in the treatment of common ailments such as constipation, asthma, sinus problems, stress, migraine and headaches, digestive disorders, back pain, bladder trouble, chronic fatigue syndrome and even more serious conditions like kidney and gall stones.

How reflexology works is not easily explained and, like auricular acupuncture (see page 172) it is difficult to comprehend how pressure applied to the feet can have therapeutic benefits in other parts of the body. But reflexologists strongly defend the technique, arguing that there is no good reason why it should not be effective.

While it is advisable that treatment for complicated or serious disorders be carried out by a trained therapist, simple techniques can be learned so that you can treat comparatively minor conditions at home. However, you will need instruction from an experienced practitioner on how and which techniques to use.

The art of foot reflexology is to apply pressure with the edge of the thumb or fingers with a circular movement, massaging the area for some minutes. Therapist sessions last 10–30 minutes but you can massage your feet as often as you like throughout the day. Approximately 10 minutes of therapy on each foot is usually sufficient to induce effective stimulation.

A foot massage is heaven for some people. They find it so soothing, enjoyable and relaxing that they fall asleep. Yet others have such sensitive feet they become quite hysterical when their feet are touched. Nevertheless, massage does not tickle and a trained reflexologist will resolve any sensitivity with appropriate techniques. Some degree of pain can be experienced when a reflex point is pressed: this can indicate a problem in the area of the body related to that particular point.

The following diagrams show the organs of the body as represented on the feet.

Some reflexology points.

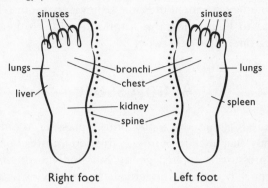

Right foot   Left foot

You can give yourself a foot massage while sitting in a comfortable chair, on the floor or in a bed with your back supported by cushions, in a warm quiet room. Rest one foot on the opposite knee and pressure can then be easily applied to the foot with both hands. Begin by massaging the whole foot with fingers and thumbs. You can then concentrate on any particular tender spots and stimulate them with gentle but firm massaging pressure; however, do not overwork these areas to the point of discomfort.

Our modern lifestyle hinders natural stimulation of the feet because we are always wearing shoes and walking on flat, even surfaces. So, even if you don't want to try reflexology, you can stimulate your feet in a very simple way. Just take off your shoes! Go barefoot in the park, walk over a variety of surfaces, wriggle your toes in the sand, or buy a pair of specially designed massage sandals. For a more general, overall reflexology stimulation even a soft drink bottle or tennis ball rolled backwards and forwards on the floor with the feet can be used.

REFLEXOLOGY AND ASTHMA
Massaging the lung area on the foot would be the best place to start for an asthma sufferer. The reflex areas in the back and sides of the smaller toes should not be ignored, for they are related to respiratory complaints such as hay fever, sinus, colds and catarrh. Other areas, such as the spine, spleen, kidney or liver, could also prove helpful. Use a circular rolling motion with the thumb and fingers, and press and massage these points.

Although we do not claim that reflexology will dramatically

improve asthma, such treatments may well be of some benefit. Michael Bradley, a patient of Ron's, believes that foot reflexology does more to help relieve his asthma than any other therapy. How does one argue otherwise?

Acupressure

Acupressure is simply the application of pressure to one or more of the many acupuncture points on the body. Instead of inserting needles, pressure is applied gently but firmly with the fingers, thumb, knuckle joints or fingernails and the point is massaged or kneaded for 5–10 seconds at a time.

Acupressure is very similar to shiatsu (see pages 155–6). It is used to relieve ailments including allergies, arthritis, asthma, digestive disorders, incontinence, insomnia, back pain, migraine, depression and tension. As with acupuncture, acupressure is believed to balance the flow of energy through the body that the Chinese call **chi** or **qi**, thus increasing the body's healing powers, preventing illness and improving vitality.

Although some pressure points may be tender when massaged, acupressure is a simple, safe and effective method for the relief of minor disorders, but it should not be relied on completely to relieve asthma and must be used in conjunction with other treatments or therapies suggested in this book. In fact most of us instinctively use acupressure to soothe a headache by pressing our hands against our foreheads. Of course, in order to use acupressure on yourself you will need to learn the correct points to apply pressure for particular ailments. There are hundreds of different points so you will need professional help to begin with.

Acupressure can be safely used at home for everyday ailments such as headaches, toothache, menstrual cramps, constipation and nausea. Do not use self-help acupressure if painful symptoms exist: consult your doctor or acupressure therapist first. More serious illnesses should be treated by a trained therapist.

The attraction of self-help acupressure is that you can repeat the massage as often as necessary; however, the routines need to be learned from a trained therapist. Some therapists suggest that while watching television or waiting at traffic lights we can help our bodies relax by applying finger and thumb pressure to the chest, especially between the ribs (intercostal bones) from the neck to the bottom of the sternum.

Acupressure points in intercostal spaces.

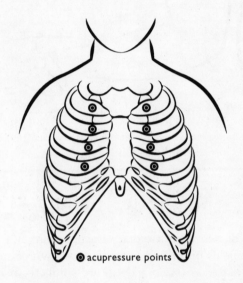

acupressure points

In recent years acupressure aids such as earrings, called "acurings," have been designed. These apply light pressure to the lung and heart points in the ear. The earrings are only worn for 20–60 minutes a day, have no known side effects and their supporters believe they assist stress, compulsive eating behavior, insomnia, excessive smoking and "nerves."

ACUPRESSURE AND ASTHMA
Activating pressure points in the cheek, nose and on various parts of the chest, back and shoulders can often help relieve asthma and act as a preventive measure. The Chinese, in particular, believe that pressure and stimulation of the lung points successfully relieves asthma and the most effective areas are located in the elbow crease and above the wrist. Acupressure to these points also helps coughs, headaches and a stiff neck. Asthma lung points are shown on the diagram overleaf.

Asthma lung points.

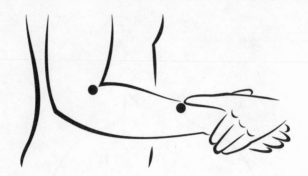

Magnetic Therapy

A synthesis of two theories, that of acupressure and the effects of magnetic fields on *chi*, magnetic therapy involves placing ball bearings or flat magnets on acupressure points to treat ailments. The magnets are held in position by adhesive tape and can be left in place for varying lengths of time, depending on the disorder being treated. They can be safely worn for many days, although it is advisable to move them slightly from time to time. They are most commonly about the size of a small pea.

Magnetic therapy is natural, painless, drugless and has no known adverse effects. Many arthritic sufferers swear by it and are adamant that it relieves their pain. However, anyone who is pregnant or wears a pacemaker should consult his or her doctor before trying this therapy.

Increasing interest in magnetic therapy has resulted in a wide range of products being developed. Magnets have been put inside body supports for the back, knees, ankles, wrist, elbows, head and neck. They have been designed to be inserted in pillows, bedding, even shoe insoles. There is magnetic jewelry, especially bracelets, which can be worn to help pain-affected areas. Many health food stores stock these products.

Jan, a 25-year-old nurse, has had two major back operations.

She is reluctant to take strong medication and her condition is such that future treatment for her is limited. Jan wears a magnet-impregnated back brace which is giving her more pain relief than anything else she has tried.

MAGNETIC THERAPY AND ASTHMA

For asthma and respiratory disorders, magnets are usually placed on acupuncture points on the sternum and along the spine.

Shiatsu

Shiatsu is a Japanese term (from **shi**, finger and **atsu**, pressure) for a stimulating massage technique used for the relief of pain or chronic stiffness and to help strengthen bones, to tone up poor circulation, the nervous and immune systems and improve the body's metabolism. It's no longer just finger pressure, though, as the thumbs, palms and heels of the hands, forearms, elbows, knees and even feet are also used to stimulate the flow of life force (*chi*) along the body's energy paths (meridians), by applying pressure to the hundreds of surface points.

Like Chinese acupressure, this safe and effective system was traditionally used as a home treatment and handed down through generations of Japanese families. Earlier this century Tokyujiro Namikoshi popularized shiatsu outside Japan, and it is now more widely used in the West than acupressure.

Shiatsu essentially aims to prevent disorders through improving general health but can also relieve a wide range of ailments, including migraine, toothache, back pain, digestive disorders, stress, depression and insomnia. Shiatsu practitioners explain that finger pressure applied to muscles in good condition will generally cause no unusual sensation. However, touching a muscle that is damaged in some way will result in an entirely different response. With finger pressure, it is often possible to restore an area of the body that is not in good condition to normal function.

Some 50 hours of training are needed before you can treat yourself and others with shiatsu, but you should only practice shiatsu at home on minor complaints. There are many approved teaching centers throughout the world, and these can supply a list of competent and qualified practitioners.

SHIATSU AND ASTHMA

Almost anyone can learn simple treatments that will relieve fatigue, aching shoulders and assist during a mild asthma attack. A lay person should only use shiatsu to help during a mild attack, though, and should cease treatment immediately if the asthma worsens. Serious attacks of asthma should be referred to a physician or a competent shiatsu practitioner.

However, shiatsu can help prevent asthma attacks. After a tiring day working, or if you are under stress, half an hour of shiatsu is not only very relaxing but regenerates the body's natural forces and improves general well-being, thus lessening the probability of asthma occurring.

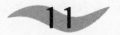

OTHER USEFUL
THERAPIES

Yoga

Yoga epitomizes the theme of this book: combining the art of relaxation with diaphragmatically controlled breathing and a positive mental attitude. Now an integral part of life for millions of people throughout the world, yoga is not simply a series of exercises but a form of complete development of both the mental and physical being.

Yoga trains the mind to develop spiritual and mental well-being, through physical movements and breathing patterns. It aims to unite the individual spirit with the universal spirit, thus giving the body added strength. Its practice does not conflict with any religious beliefs but contributes to and intensifies spiritual awareness, thereby helping the forces of the body in their role of restoration and healing.

Since its origin in India some 3000 years ago, various forms of yoga have developed, each having its own particular philosophy and movements. Recently Western society has enthusiastically taken up the physical hatha system as a means of cleansing

the body of impurities, reducing weight, toning and stimulating
the nervous system, strengthening muscles and generally improving health. Other yoga traditions have different aims: raja yoga
focuses on mind control; jnana yoga concentrates on intellect
and understanding; karma yoga encourages service to others;
bhakti yoga emphasizes devotion and care; and mantra yoga is
mainly concerned with vibrations and radiations of life. The
various philosophies do take a great deal of study and the general
understanding of them in the West is very limited.

Hatha yoga's basic concept is to extend the physical body
to its natural limits, develop breath control and thus to intensify
self control, cultivate mind and body coordination, tap the inner
sources of the body, strengthen muscles and expand the immune
system. Supporters believe it prolongs life. While yoga can be
practiced by all ages, those around middle age seem to practice
it most enthusiastically. Perhaps their maturity allows them a
greater understanding of the philosophy.

It is not the purpose of this book to explain particular yoga
techniques but we do encourage you to consider trying yoga.
Yoga schools are found all around the world. If you don't have
a school convenient to you, numerous books and videos are
available explaining the philosophy and breathing techniques,
and illustrating the poses, postures, movements and exercises.

YOGA AND ASTHMA

Yoga results in improved physical strength, breathing control and
mental health, which are vital contributors to improving an asthmatic condition. Yoga teachers everywhere will give evidence of
cases where yoga has helped those suffering from asthma.

Debra, one of Ron's patients, had suffered from asthma for
many years. She tried yoga and was so impressed with its effectiveness she is now a full-time teacher of the technique. She
insists yoga is the major reason she is now completely asthma-
free.

If only for the breathing technique, hatha yoga will unques-
tionably provide you with skills to help control and alleviate your
asthma. However, as your health improves through mastering
your body you will probably want to progress to higher stages
of training – which will ultimately bring you to greater self-
awareness, inner peace, happiness and joie de vivre.

T'ai-chi

During a recent visit to China to study acupuncture further, Ron watched enviously every morning as hundreds of people practiced the art of t'ai-chi before beginning their daily tasks. The slow, passive, dance-like movements being performed in parklands and open spaces by so many people looked so graceful and simple that Ron wanted to join them in this peaceful pursuit and eagerly sought classes on his return. T'ai-chi is now becoming a routine for millions of people in the Western world too. Although a highly complex form of exercise, it is not merely a work-out, but a complete, natural and effective therapy focusing on mental, emotional and physical harmony.

T'ai-chi, meaning "wholeness," is an abbreviation of the Chinese **t'ai-chi ch'uan**, meaning "supreme, ultimate." It was first practiced by Taoist monks in the fourteenth century, with the aim of mastering the self, mind and body harmony in motion.

T'ai-chi's smooth, easy flowing movements – likened to those of birds and animals – encourage body awareness through a physical routine of relaxation, controlled breathing, flexibility and mobility. Although requiring patience and perseverance to learn, t'ai-chi replaces stress, anxiety, aggression and hostility with calmness, serenity, sensitivity and peace. T'ai-chi unfolds its benefits gradually and requires regular attendance at classes to learn the many movements. A short form of t'ai-chi has been developed recently, with about 40 nonrepetitive movements, but this does not have quite the therapeutic value of the hundred or so actions of the traditional version.

Many organizations and centers conduct regular classes and much more detailed information about t'ai-chi can be had from local community groups, libraries or telephone books.

Chi

Traditional Chinese philosophy talks a great deal about **chi** or **qi**, an innate energy force or power flowing through the body which encourages and stimulates all living creatures. T'ai-chi is based on the belief that illness stems from **chi** moving too slowly or too quickly, resulting in imbalances of energy in particular areas of the body. For example, if too much energy is in the head and chest and too little in the legs, the body becomes "top-heavy" and this needs to be corrected by mentally focusing on the correct **chi** through the performance of various movements.

Many Westerners have great difficulty in understanding the concept of **chi**, but have experienced its power when a needle was inserted in an acupuncture point in their body. Stimulating **chi** produces a hyped-up feeling, as if from adrenalin running through the body. The sensation is almost impossible to describe, but an auto mechanic explained it as "the feeling you get when you touch a spark plug;" it has been likened by others to the static electricity from nylon. Experiences of **chi** vary from person to person but the ultimate effect is one of energy rippling through the body just like the expanding, rippling circle caused by throwing a stone into a pond.

T'AI-CHI AND ASTHMA

Eliminating anxiety and stress, developing controlled diaphragmatic breathing and relaxation techniques, toning up the body and stimulating the circulation are t'ai-chi's aims, and are just what this book is all about too. T'ai-chi can provide all these elements in the quest for asthma relief and good health.

Feldenkrais Technique

Moshe Feldenkrais, a Russian-born Israeli trained in engineering and applied physics, was involved in France's atomic program and British antisubmarine research. One of the first Europeans to become a black belt in judo, Feldenkrais devised movements to teach people about their body's machinery. He believed that the body is arranged to move with minimum effort and maximum efficiency but that the brain's images of the correct pattern of movement become scrambled and the result is the brain instructs the body to move incorrectly and painfully.

Feldenkrais formulated two techniques to undo this misinformation. Awareness Through Movement aims to make people aware of their inappropriate habitual patterns and to correct them through movements taught in classes. Functional Integration, which is conducted on a one-to-one basis, achieves the same results with gentle manipulation.

Feldenkrais classes lead students through sequences of gentle movements or rotations, repeated until they become smooth, rhythmic and easy to perform. These movements are not strenuous but usually involve opposite movements, such as turning the head to the right at the same time as turning the left shoulder and upper torso in the opposite direction.

FELDENKRAIS TECHNIQUE AND ASTHMA

Asthmatics often have a stooped posture, with round shoulders and an inverted chest. Good posture is essential for good breathing, and therefore for asthmatics. The Feldenkrais technique (along with the Alexander technique, yoga and t'ai-chi) provides a valuable avenue to rectify poor body structure.

Any exercise regimen or therapy which fully extends the body's range of muscles, tendons and ligaments gently, slowly and methodically releasing stress and producing a relaxed physical and mental attitude, is ideal for asthma sufferers.

Here is a spine-flexing back exercise based on the Feldenkrais technique that is particularly helpful in improving upper back posture and thus alleviating asthma. Sit upright in a chair, cross your right leg over your left leg and with your left hand grasp your right foot and pull it towards you. At the same time rotate the upper part of your body fully to the right as far as you can go and hold for 2–3 seconds. Slowly return to the starting position. Repeat 6–8 times. Change position and cross the left leg over the right leg, grasp the foot with the right hand and pull it towards you. Then rotate the body to the left, hold for 2–3 seconds, return slowly to starting position and repeat 6–8 times. These movements should be done gently and smoothly, breathing **out** slowly from the diaphragm and letting breathing in just happen automatically.

Alexander Technique

Aldous Huxley, the author of *Brave New World*, wrote:

The Alexander Technique can give us all the things that we have been looking for in a system of physical education: relief from strain due to maladjustment and constant improvement in physical and mental health. You cannot ask more from any system; nor if we seriously desire to alter human beings in a desirable direction, can we ask less.

F. Matthias Alexander, an actor and reciter of poetry and humorous pieces, was born in Australia in 1869. As a result of bouts of hoarseness which affected his theatrical performances, Alexander made a study of muscular contractions in and around his neck and head. He discovered that his stage posture put pressure on his vocal cords, tightened his throat, interfered with his breathing and created tension throughout his body. By correcting and learning from his own postural imperfections, he developed a technique of teaching people to unlearn harmful and unnatural postures and retrain the body's movements and positions. Alexander's watchword was "Health, health, health."

The Alexander technique encourages self-awareness and the relationship and harmony of mind and body. Successful treatment claims have been made for many ailments including high blood pressure, respiratory disorders, irritable bowel syndrome, colitis, rheumatoid arthritis, osteoarthritis, back pain, sciatica and asthma. Asthma-related disorders such as unnatural curvature of the spine can also be assisted by this technique.

Although intended as a self-help method, the Alexander technique needs to be taught by a qualified practitioner who will identify your problems and show you how to change harmful postures. Lessons last about 30–45 minutes and, depending on your condition, you may require a course of up to 30 sessions to completely master the technique.

A simple self-help starting point is to watch yourself in a mirror while standing, walking or sitting. Do you stand with more weight on one leg, hip thrown out to the side? Do you walk with your head down and shoulders stooped? Do you slouch in a chair? By constantly being aware of your poor posture you can think about and practice good posture all the time. As you stand, think about trying to touch the ceiling with the top of your head and stretch your neck and back out towards it. Learn to use your body correctly and release the tension: walk tall, stand tall.

ALEXANDER TECHNIQUE AND ASTHMA

Recent scientific research has confirmed Alexander's views about natural posture, health and the connection between anxiety and physical tension. Asthmatics in particular must think of their posture if they want to improve their breathing, and their health.

Hydrotherapy

Hydrotherapy covers a number of healing modalities, for it means "healing using water." However, many current ideas can be traced back to Sebastian Kneipp (1821–97), a Dominican monk from Bavaria who is the recognized founder of modern hydrotherapy.

Author of books on the healing benefits of water, Kneipp cured himself of a lung disorder by a routine of plunging himself into ice-cold water, then warming himself with vigorous exercise. He recommended walking barefoot in wet grass and cold streams, which would stimulate a resurgence of blood to the limbs, creating warmth naturally and activating the body's own healing powers. Many of his treatments were adopted by naturopaths. His ideas have been extended to include natural spring waters, whirlpools, underwater massage and, more recently, flotation tanks and aqua-aerobics.

Spas have always been places of pilgrimage for the sick. It is an extremely therapeutic and relaxing experience to spend some time in the waters of natural mineral springs or spas, and people with a variety of complaints benefit from the water. Exercising in a heated pool, for instance, is one of the best ways to reduce the stiffness and pain of arthritic joints and improve muscle tone. The relaxing warmth and buoyancy of the water makes exercising pleasurable rather than painful.

Fundamentally, water is the essence of life. It is the substance that makes up the major part of our bodies, and of our foods. We can only live a few days without it. For healing, however, the most significant aspect of water is its temperature. Cold water applications constrict blood vessels, reduce surface inflammation and congestion and stimulate the flow of blood to the internal organs. Steam from hot water dilates blood vessels, encourages sweating, and relaxes muscles and joints.

Many different forms of treatment are offered by professional and qualified naturopaths and physiotherapists, but depending on the nature of your condition simple hydrotherapy can be used at home. Alternate the temperature of your daily shower from hot to cold, finishing with cold and have a brisk rub down with a towel: this will improve circulation and make your body glow.

Adding epsom salts (magnesium sulphate) and a teaspoon of eucalyptus oil or appropriate essential oil (see pages 133–7) to a warm bath provides your body with much needed minerals and helps drive off colds and chills. Fifteen minutes soaking in the enriched water is about all you need to relax and soothe you all over. Likewise, soaking your feet in a foot bath with epsom salts added, followed by a foot massage, is a wonderfully relaxing experience. Or there is the latest in luxury appliances to help you feel good – mini spa baths for the feet!

Steam inhalations with refreshing oils such as eucalyptus, lavender, wintergreen or thyme effectively clear nasal passages and relieve congestion, catarrh, asthma, croup and whooping cough and improve skin conditions such as acne by opening facial pores and sweating out impurities.

Saunas or sweat baths using eucalyptus or other essential oils relieve colds, flu, catarrh or bronchial conditions and may even alleviate an asthma attack. Of course, a sauna or sweat bath should be followed by a tepid bath or shower to lower the body temperature gradually and avoid catching a chill.

In flotation tanks, the latest innovation in the realm of hydrotherapy, common salt (sodium chloride) is used not only to soothe aching muscles but also to support the patient's body-weight, making flotation more comfortable. Flotation tanks often have built-in motivational tapes playing, or calming relaxing music, to heighten the enjoyment of this recreational experience.

HYDROTHERAPY AND ASTHMA

A relaxed body responds positively to healing, a tense body rejects it. People with asthma should not underestimate hydrotherapy when looking for ways to reduce the anxiety and stress of their condition and improve their overall health. Inhalations may also help significantly in clearing the air passages, so should be tried by people with asthma.

Reiki

Reiki is a healing system that originated in Japan, where it has been practiced for centuries. It reached the West through the teaching of Dr. Mikao Usui in the first half of this century. The Usui system of reiki is an ancient holistic method of treating the mind, body and soul. Reiki uses the "universal life force" that followers believe surrounds us, by transmitting its energy to mobilize the body's healing resources into reversing disease. Reiki's "energy work" attempts to accelerate the body's ability to heal itself and correct the imbalances which lead to disease.

This nonintrusive therapy is deeply relaxing but at the same time energizing. It is said to recognize the source of a problem and address it directly. In the course of a treatment there is a rebalancing effect on the chakras of the body, which can purify the energy flow within the body – thus making it more resistant to disease and disorders – and loosen any energy blocks. The chakras are a concept without a good equivalent in Western tradition, and can perhaps loosely be described as the places within the body that are the focuses of the body's internal energy flow.

Reiki energy is channelled through the practitioner's hands and is described by most people as a warm or tingling sensation. Specific hand positions are held over various areas of the body for several minutes and an average treatment may last 60–90 minutes. The overall physical experience is generally felt as a gentle but deeply relaxing warmth.

Whether or not you accept that universal life energy can accelerate healing, you may find reiki helpful. Reiki is used to heal many disorders, stress-related illnesses and injuries. During the last 20 years, the rapid spread of reiki throughout the Western world has led to more orthodox professions using it as a support therapy. Basic reiki classes start with self-treatment techniques and, after some months practice, lead to advanced level courses. Its self-help facet is valuable for those who might be reluctant to depend on others for a complementary healing therapy to improve their vitality.

Ron experienced reiki in a way unconnected with asthma. He found himself sitting opposite a reiki practitioner at a dinner. When she asked Ron if he had any current ailments, he admitted to a constantly painful big toe. She asked Ron to take his shoe off and she then held his foot for 20 minutes or so. To Ron's surprise, the pain disappeared and he had no sign of it again for a considerable time. Such a story is common among people who have experienced reiki: you do not have to be a "believer" in order for reiki to have an effect.

Note   Reiki must not be confused with Reichian Therapy (also known as Orgone Therapy), which is explained in Chapter 14, "Some Esoteric Therapies and Techniques."

REIKI AND ASTHMA

Reiki practitioners believe that when stress is the underlying cause of asthma, asthmatics should use reiki and good stress management techniques to help them lessen the likelihood of attacks.

Therapeutic Touch

In Anglo-Saxon societies we shake hands when we meet, in other societies people greet acquaintances with a kiss on the cheek. Some cultures rub noses. These are natural ways of "breaking the ice" and getting to know someone. Cuddling a baby, holding hands on a date, nursing a sick person, hugging and kissing, are all examples of the need to touch.

Touch is vital to relationships between human beings. We all feel better when we are loved, touched and comforted. Touching puts us at peace with one another and with ourselves.

It is considered a privilege for someone to be allowed to enter the boundaries of another's aura. And, if you think about it, we've all reacted unfavorably at some time to personal intrusion. How often have we resisted the initial touch of someone and felt uncomfortable if they invade "our" space?

Small children have no sense of personal space, but as adolescence is reached a feeling grows of a volume that belongs to the individual, one that others may only be invited to enter. Unfortunately some people develop very strong barriers to their space and are not at ease touching another person. They are usually very tense, anxiety-driven people who always seem to have something wrong with them.

Such people must recognize that it is not an invasion of space when someone comes close to show they care. Learning to let go, relax, and allow people into the space occasionally will lessen the barriers. The results will be the disappearance of those feelings of uneasiness around other people, and the restoration of well-being.

Even the simple act of shaking hands can create a state of trust, break down barriers, establish friendship, present a feeling of warmth, offer solace or congratulations. Patting someone on the head is a gesture of approval for a young person, while holding the hand of someone who is ill is comforting and relaxing to the patient.

Hands can be sensitive to a person's needs and both the receiver and the giver can feel nurtured and harmonized by being touched. We can use our personal "laying on of hands" in many ways to make someone feel better. Healing accelerates when we know someone cares about us and we are not alone.

We all need to be touching and touched for health – give someone a hug today.

Chi and touching

Brushing over and along the **chi**'s meridian pathways is an ancient Chinese custom believed to pass one person's energies to another. With feather-like strokes, both hands brush very, very lightly in one direction along acupuncture meridian pathways. This touching and giving of care and energy is said to reduce blockages, energize **chi**, activate the body's healing mechanism and balance the aura. Brushing restores balance and harmony in the body and is a safe support therapy to promote well-being and a relaxed frame of mind and body.

Laying on of hands

Healers throughout the world have been trying for thousands of years to cure people by nonphysical means. Clearly there are many possible methods, but the "laying on of hands" is one many people recognize. A fundamental part of the early Christian church, which is still practiced today, the laying on of hands, or hand healing, is supposed to use the healer to transmit divine healing power.

Spiritual healers believe that a divine source channels healing powers through them to increase the patient's healing and make him or her whole. Many religious and healing "laying on of hands" experiences are well documented and it is not uncommon to read that one has resulted in pain lessening, tension easing and waves of energy sweeping through afflicted areas. The healing potential of this simple act may defy scientific understanding – but who can really say it doesn't work or explain why it does?

Hand healers explain that a healing force exists that can be tapped for healing purposes and this force can be channelled through individuals into people in need. In many ways laying on of hands is similar to reiki. Practitioners claim the healing force does not need any faith on the part of the patient to work. This is not to say healers dismiss the faith factor or the psychological aspect of their healing that may be working through hypnosis or autosuggestion.

A healer concentrates his or her attention on the affected area, either while touching it with his fingers or palms of his hands, or with his hands on the patient's head. The patient often feels sensations being transmitted from the hands as healing energies enter his or her aura.

Auras – luminous areas of light with misty outlines – are believed to surround people, animals, plants and sometimes even inanimate objects. Kirlian high-frequency photography has captured on film auras around the fingers of healers when they are healing someone.

Kirlian photography is a technique developed by a Russian husband-and-wife team, Semyon and Valentina Kirlian. Semyon observed flashes of light between electrodes and the skin when he visited a research institute in Europe. The Kirlians began experimenting with photographing and illuminating subjects using alternating currents of high frequency. After 40 years of experimental photography in relative obscurity, the Kirlians' results were published. Their many and varied photographs of hands, feet, flowers, and plants revealed a luminescence – an aura – beyond the outline of the living things. The auras proved, they believed, that a "life force" (sometimes called a bioplanic energy) existed. Kirlian photography produces prints of auras and, by examining these, the subject's state of health can be determined and diseases diagnosed before any outward symptoms are displayed. High-frequency photography has been used for some 20 years in what used to be the Soviet Union, but the West has not practiced it as a diagnostic tool quite as readily.

More recent studies have revealed auras around such inanimate objects as earrings, brooches, coins, etc., which rather dispels the theory that a life force only exists in organic substances. Whatever Kirlian photography is capturing on film, it appears there may be something present around objects that healers refer to as the healing force. If so it may also be true that the force can be used by a healer's hands.

However laying on of hands works, countless people worldwide do believe in its efficacy; the scientific and medical professions are still skeptical.

THERAPEUTIC TOUCH AND ASTHMA

A severe attack of asthma doesn't seem so bad when a caring person is nearby to touch and comfort us. Touching is calming, and some asthma attacks will recede if the patient calms. However, you should not rely on touch, or hand healing, to prevent asthma or to halt an attack.

TREATMENTS AND DEVICES

Acupuncture

Acupuncture is not suitable for children.

Acupuncture is the practice of inserting very fine needles, generally stainless steel, into one of many hundreds of points on the body – including some 250 points in the ear. These points lie along the "meridians," or energy channels of the body, and are said to be linked to specific internal organs. Acupuncture has been used in China, Korea and Japan for over 2000 years but it has only become popular this century in Western countries. However it is now used to treat a wide variety of diseases and complaints – asthma being one of the more successful.

The Chinese believe that a life force, **chi** or **qi**, flows through the body and that acupuncture stimulates this energy at particular points on the body. The flow of **chi** is believed to be unblocked, decreased or increased by the needles.

There are 14 meridians flowing vertically through the body, passing through the major organs – spleen, kidneys, stomach, liver, bladder, lungs, heart and so on – and the meridians are named after a particular organ. However, points along the meridians are used to treat disorders other than those affecting the named organ. Modern acupuncture charts show up to 2000 treatment points along the meridians, although traditional Chinese medicine only indicated 365.

The Chinese consider good health to be a state of balance and harmony, and that in everything that lives there is an interaction between two polar energy forces: yin and yang. There is no absolute yin and no absolute yang, only a mixture of the two, although the balance may swing. Neither can exist without the other – they are constantly interacting and changing. Acupuncture maintains the harmonious balance of yin and yang in the body by stimulating or sedating the energy flow, thereby equalizing the forces and allowing nature to restore the body to good health. Yang organs in the body are the denser organs and include the heart, liver, spleen, kidneys and lungs. The yin organs are the more hollow organs, such as the large and small intestines, the gall bladder and the stomach.

Acupuncture is a quick, painless and bloodless procedure. There is just a slight numbness or tingling sensation where the needle is inserted. The needles are very fine (0.25–0.5 mm in diameter) and vary in length from 1 cm to 5 cm. The treatment can vary considerably from one consultation to another and for some complaints as many as 20 needles can be used at one time. The needles remain inserted for 25–30 minutes.

The acupuncture points are generally nerve endings. An electrical stimulus in the form of leads operating from a low-voltage acupuncture stimulator can be attached to the needles, which speeds up the effects of acupuncture. This current eliminates the need to vibrate the needles by hand, the traditional way to stimulate the flow of **chi**. The stimulatory effect of acupuncture reaches a peak about 10 minutes from inserting the needle and then slowly recedes during the next 10–15 minutes.

When needles are inserted in an acupuncture point, endorphins (the body's natural hormonal pain-killers) are aroused so acupuncture is often used, especially in the West, to treat painful conditions such as arthritis, back pain and rheumatism. It has also successfully helped people suffering from asthma, allergies, angina, anxiety, bronchitis, colitis, digestive and gallbladder problems, insomnia, stress, tiredness and ulcers.

Skepticism and fear of needles often deter people from the healing potential of acupuncture but any apprehension is soon dispelled during a first treatment. Perhaps surprisingly, most people look forward to further visits.

Auricular acupuncture – acupuncture in and around the ear – is a related healing technique. It is often more effective than body acupuncture. Auricular points may also be used in the treatment of asthma. A recent development has been acupuncture of the nose, hands and feet, in which there are also numerous points to help an asthmatic condition.

Qualified, competent acupuncturists are established in major cities throughout the world. It is absolutely essential that you consult a practitioner who belongs to a reputable organization. You should ensure the acupuncturist has received formal training and educational qualifications and adheres to a strict professional code of ethics and practice. Needles inserted incorrectly can cause serious harm. **Under no circumstances should you allow an unqualified person to administer acupuncture to you**.

Stringent licensing conditions now ensure that acupuncture treatments' hygiene and cleanliness meet with the approval of appropriate health authorities. Because of the danger of blood-borne infection being passed between patients, reusable needles must be sterilized in an autoclave machine. Nowadays the widespread use of disposable acupuncture needles in sealed, sterilized packs has reduced the risk of contamination.

ACUPUNCTURE AND ASTHMA

Because asthma is a chronic condition, it is not easy to say specifically that acupuncture will remedy it, except that numerous studies and thousands of case histories worldwide convincingly demonstrate its success. Acute attacks have been relieved when sedative points are activated to relax the asthmatic, but asthma is more likely to improve if the acupuncture is given when an attack is not in progress, the treatment being aimed instead at strengthening the lungs and prevention. The lung, stomach and large intestine meridians are most frequently used to treat asthma.

Acupuncture promotes a relaxed state of mind, which in turn activates the healing mechanism, and people with asthma usually start feeling better within about four to six sessions. However, such a complex medical condition may need more sessions before there is a clear improvement.

Marion Adams, one of Ron's patients, strongly believes that acupuncture has been instrumental in relieving her asthma. Like many others, Marion finds it difficult to explain why and how acupuncture works but is emphatic that it is effective for her.

Another patient, Jack Carless, suffered severely from bronchitis and asthma. As he was approaching seventy his condition was expected to deteriorate; however, Jack learned Controlled Pattern Breathing and had acupuncture. As a result his health improved dramatically. Jack has acupuncture on a monthly basis and looks forward to the wonderful feeling of relaxation and lightness he experiences from the energy flow through his body.

Laser Acupuncture

Possibly the most innovative, effective and noninvasive method of applying heat to acupuncture points, laser acupuncture is now often used instead of acupuncture needles. For children and people who are afraid of needles laser acupuncture is a more suitable method of treatment than traditional acupuncture. The range of complaints that can be treated by laser acupuncture is identical to needle acupuncture.

Laser acupuncture sends a beam of light from a laser tube down on to an acupuncture point, and the light stimulates the point in the same way a needle would. The only visible sign is the red beam radiated from the helium and neon gases, "heating" the acupuncture point. The beam is held in position for a minimum of 10 seconds and a maximum of two minutes, depending on the amount of tissue to be penetrated and the power applied. Infrared lasers (which do not have any visible light beam, but work in the same way) are also used. When laser acupuncture is being practiced around the face, patients wear protective glasses to screen their eyes from the beam.

There are reports that the feeling of **chi** is less apparent during laser acupuncture than when needles are inserted into the acupuncture points. However, the latest research indicates laser therapy is just as effective as needle acupuncture and patients who have experienced both seem divided over which they prefer.

Most people say that no matter which method is used, the results are more than satisfactory.

Laser acupuncture is gradually becoming more common as an increasing number of acupuncturists train to administer it. If you are offered laser acupuncture you can be sure it is safe: government bodies exercise close control over the use of laser equipment and manufacturers must meet stringent safety standards.

Electrical Massagers

Electrical massagers are not suitable for children.

A variety of electrical massagers have been designed to help relax or stimulate the body. As long as the stimulation is not excessive and is only for about 5–10 minutes, it is unlikely that a mechanical or electrical massager will cause any harm.

Chiropractic patients are usually given mild to moderate massage before adjustments, by hand or with an electrical massager on and around the spinal column. However, massage is not given if the patient has a fever, blood poisoning, acute inflammation, skin disease, abscesses, hemorrhage, spinal disease, tubercular joints, heart condition, is menstruating or pregnant or has severe abdominal pain.

ELECTRICAL MASSAGERS AND ASTHMA

Controlled vibration for a short time on the back, especially in the ribcage area (thorax), can be of great benefit for an asthma sufferer. If you buy an electrical massager to help your asthma at home, you will, of course, need someone to apply the massager for you. Massage should be given on the back and shoulders only, with the clothes on or over a towel, not directly on the skin and never during an asthma attack. The massage pressure should be comfortable, not painful, and the operator should be careful not to press too hard.

Regular massage is very relaxing as long as it is at a tolerable level. Massage should give you pleasure and relief, and can ease the tension in the upper body so often experienced by people with asthma.

Transcutaneous Nerve Stimulation

Transcutaneous nerve stimulation is not suitable for children.

A transcutaneous nerve stimulator (TNS) is a small battery-powered machine which sends extremely weak electrical impulses through the skin via a pair of rubber pads to activate the nerves that block out pain. The concept is not new, but the machine is. Originally a Roman doctor placed a patient's swollen foot on a live electric eel to treat gout! When it became possible to store static electricity, doctors in the nineteenth century relieved various aches and pains by sending electric currents through patients' bodies. Dentists did likewise to ease the pain of tooth extraction. Thankfully progress has modernized electrical nerve stimulation. TNS may be given in hospitals and doctors' offices, but there are also small, hand-held (although less effective) TNS appliances that can be attached to a specific point on the body and switched on at any time.

Designed primarily for the treatment of lumbago, sciatica and sports injuries, TNS machines are also effective as a drug alternative for nonpainful circulation problems. When turned to high-frequency mode, TNS operates as a pain block, and many hospital maternity wards have specifically designed TNS machines to reduce the pain of childbirth. New types of machine automatically vary their pulsing rate, depending on the part of the body being treated.

Busy "hands-on" therapists can set up a TNS machine and leave a patient quietly on his own for 5–10 minutes to enjoy a mild pulsing and relaxing massage from the low-voltage induced vibration.

TNS AND ASTHMA

Applying TNS to the first and second thoracic vertebrae (see diagram on page 141) and around the scapular region (the shoulder blades), helps an asthmatic by relieving muscular tension in this area, improving the blood supply and lessening fatigue. The gentle vibration acts very much like a massage and can be used two or three times per day for 5–10 minutes at a time.

TNS machines can be borrowed or rented from some hospitals or medical suppliers. Proper instruction is essential to know where the pads should be placed and how to operate the machine. A TNS machine should **not** be used by people with heart pacemakers as it can interfere with the pacemaker's performance.

Magneton Therapy or Bioenergetic Acupuncture

You will have learned at school about the earth's magnetic field and the pull of the North and South Poles. And, like most of us, you probably have not thought too much about it since. But perhaps magnetic therapy can improve asthma.

Magneton therapy is currently having quite an impact, being used to treat a variety of ailments, from various respiratory conditions to painful conditions, as well as fatigue, dizziness, eating disorders, and insomnia. Remarkable success has been achieved with magneton therapy to relieve painful muscular disorders and disease involving the nerves, skin, blood vessels and bones.

An explanation of how magneton therapy works is that because blood contains iron ions in its hemoglobin, the iron in the blood will be attracted to magnetic fields, and hence magnetic fields applied to the body will rapidly increase blood flow and circulation. The magneton therefore allows faster restoration of normal body functions and healing processes.

Nervous vibrations surrounding and affecting the body are said to be biomagnetic and referred to as "charged batteries." Based on the knowledge that electric currents (nerve impulses) flow through the body between cell surfaces, it is believed that magnetic fields can influence the nervous system.

Magneton therapy or bioenergetic acupuncture replaces the more traditional needles with magnetic fields, to re-establish the body's energy circuits or **chi**. Used by many natural therapists and chiropractors, the magneton, or Needleless Magneton, a 1979 invention developed by Dr. Zeydel, is about the size of a matchbox. Gentle but powerful radiation from an inner core stimulates or sedates acupuncture points on which the magneton is placed. Cellular tissue is thus energized and the body's metabolism balanced.

Magneton therapy is preferred by some to traditional acupuncture as it eliminates possible problems connected with skin puncture or penetration and, of course, there is no pain.

Not a great deal of research has been conducted on the therapeutic capacity of magnetic therapy but there are vast numbers of personal testimonials to its effectiveness. It would seem it has had most success in treating muscular–skeletal problems, rheumatism and arthritis, bronchitis and asthma.

There are many other magnetic products on the market designed to be worn on acupressure points, but these are not the same as magneton therapy. You can read more about these products in Chapter 10.

Cupping

Cupping is not suitable for children.

Dating back to early Egyptian times, cupping has been used to treat a range of ailments including asthma. The Chinese, for whom cupping was also a popular remedy, theorized that it rid the body of unwanted or perverse **chi** by drawing it to the surface and diffusing it. Traditional Chinese medicine still uses cupping to treat asthma, as well as boils or abscesses, arthritis, rheumatism, bruising, colds and chills.

There are two types of cupping, wet and dry. Dry cupping is by far the most common and involves heating the air in glass or bamboo suction cups and then placing the cups along energy meridian lines or affected areas of the body. To heat the air cotton wool soaked in alcohol is ignited and held at the mouth of the cup, causing the air inside to expand. The cup is then placed mouth down on the body and as it cools the air contracts and the resulting drop in pressure in the cup draws the flesh upwards. This increases the blood flow to the surface, drawing out impurities. The cup remains in place for 4–5 minutes and is removed by exerting pressure on the skin around it to gently break the suction.

The same procedure is followed for wet cupping but shallow

cuts are then made in the raised skin, drawing blood into it and the cup applied again. Wet cupping may have been widely used years ago but would not be an acceptable technique for today's society, in view of the risk of contamination.

Recently, cups with an outlet valve that use a suction pump to draw out the air were developed. These are just as effective as the more conventional cups but eliminate the danger of the open flame and the risk of excessive heat burning the skin.

Cupping and moxibustion (see next section) should only be carried out by experienced practitioners, with the strictest sterile precautions and hygienic conditions. Cupping is not an appropriate treatment for anyone who is nervous or suffers convulsions and should not be used on skin that is ulcerated or broken.

Moxibustion

Moxibustion is not suitable for children.

Moxibustion applies localized heat to improve the body's flow of vital energy, **chi**, and treats similar ailments to cupping. Moxibustion is often used in conjunction with acupuncture.

Moxibustion is the process of placing an ignited moxa stick (a stick made from the finely powdered leaves of *Artemisia vulgaris* or mugwort) as close as possible above a specific acupuncture point. This can be done by inserting an acupuncture needle into the designated point, then placing small cones of moxa on the needle and igniting them. The heat is allowed to penetrate the skin for about 3–5 minutes or until it becomes too hot for the patient. Alternatively a small cone or roll of paper filled with moxa is ignited and the glowing tip positioned safely above the skin until it becomes hot; the cone is then removed. This process is repeated at short intervals.

As a result of our multicultural society, this ancient Eastern medicine concept has gained acceptance in the Western world, but is mostly used by Chinese practitioners – who may recommend it for treating asthma. The same precautions mentioned in cupping are relevant to moxibustion.

Air Ionizers and Purifiers

Electrically charged particles are called ions. Ions are positive or negative and we come in contact with them all the time. The air is full of ionized particles.

Ions can have a dramatic effect on our well-being. Have you ever felt irritable, depressed, tense or had a headache before a storm? Do you know why? Because positive ions fill the air before a storm and build tension. After the storm do you feel invigorated? Yes, because negative ions fill the air. Does being near clear running streams, waterfalls, in a rain forest, by the seaside, out in the sun uplift and exhilarate you? Why? Again because there are lots of negative ions in the atmosphere! Fresh seaside and mountain air is rich in negative particles, whereas city air contains few ions and any negative ions that might be around are quickly destroyed by pollution, central heating, air conditioning, electrical appliances, synthetic fibers and dust.

Environments low in negative ions or high positive-ion weather conditions like dry, hot winds sap our energy, make us feel tired and depressed and can trigger an attack of asthma or hay fever. We can be affected in the home, too, where the air's ionic balance is altered by television screens, radiators, radios, fluorescent tubes, gas heaters, nylon carpet and microwave ovens.

Ionizing machines produce a constant flow of negative ions. Small ionizers, with a range of 3–5 meters, can be plugged in near a bed or placed on a work desk or bench. More powerful units can be used in offices and larger areas. Ionization also cleans the air of allergy-causing bacteria, cigarette smoke, pollen and dust that can irritate the respiratory tract. Sufferers from asthma, bronchitis, hay fever and catarrh gain considerable relief by regular nighttime use of a bedside ionizer. A negative-ion rich environment also seems to help headaches, migraine, insomnia, depression and skin allergies. Recent studies showed that an increase in negative ions in the atmosphere may speed the healing process of wounds, sores and injuries.

Research by Dr. Leslie Hawkins at the University of Surrey, U.K., showed that levels of the hormone serotonin in the blood, brain and other tissues seemed to be reduced by negative ions. Serotonin is a substance that plays a part in brain chemistry, and imbalances in it lead to depression and other mental disturbances.

Dr. Hawkins suggested that air rich in negative ions has a stimulating effect, while too many positive ions, and thus high levels of serotonin in the body, are depressing. This may explain why ionizers help in cases of irritability and stress.

Russia, a leader in the field of ionization therapy, and Germany use negative ionizers on a public scale. There is a mass of scientific and medical evidence about the beneficial effect of negative ion therapy from all over the world. Major research done by NASA's Molecular Biophysics Laboratory showed that performance, work capacity, allergic conditions, pains, healing and burn recovery were all improved in negatively ionized air.

Small, inexpensive ionizers are now available from pharmacies, health food outlets and electrical stores. Surfaces around the ionizers need to be cleaned regularly to avoid discoloration from the matter they attract.

AIR IONIZERS AND ASTHMA

Asthmatics and hay fever sufferers who live in highly polluted areas, surrounded by electrical appliances, high tech equipment and power lines, are constantly exposed to positive ions. We believe negative ionizers will definitely help their condition.

Many natural therapists use ionizers in their homes and recommend them to patients to correct atmospheric and environmental imbalances and increase the flow of negative ions. One respected researcher, James Wright, Ph.D., has practiced traditional Western medicine for over 35 years. He is recognized for his acceptance and recommendation of hypnotherapy, acupuncture, hydrotherapy, spinal manipulation, vitamin and mineral therapy and other "fringe" modalities. Dr. Wright writes: "My evaluation indicates that ingesting small negative ions can provide significant health benefits."

Air purifiers

Fan-forced air purifiers usually contain three-way activated carbon (charcoal) filters to purify the atmosphere. Now on the market worldwide, these appliances vary in size to cover a wide range of industrial and commercial applications. Heavy industrial air purifiers can protect workers from the damaging effects of harmful chemicals, while other models purify the air in offices, classrooms, clinics and hospitals. Some purifiers also allow an air ionizer to be built in.

Air purifiers not only provide clean fresh air but also have therapeutic benefits for people affected by asthma, sinus, hay fever or respiratory disorders. Fragrant essential oils can be added to the purifier: their vapors are diffused by the fan and distributed throughout the room, refreshing the air for those with asthma, coughs, colds and nasal congestion.

Aromatherapy product companies promote small models as alternatives to oil burners. As they have no naked flame, air purifiers can be left running unattended, particularly in a child's bedroom. The constant faint aroma of eucalyptus in particular, or essential oils such as wintergreen, menthol, lavender or camphor, wafting throughout your home has valuable preventive properties. However, you should ensure the amount of essential oil used is not excessive.

AIR PURIFIERS AND ASTHMA

Air purifiers significantly reduce pollutants in the atmosphere. Anything that will rid the environment of dust, pollens, fumes, tobacco smoke, cooking smells, mildew, airborne particles and the like will reduce potential asthma triggers and thus help people with asthma.

Diagnostic Devices

Bioelectronic regulatory techniques (BER)

The idea behind these is that electrical activity in the body can be measured by bioelectronic regulatory techniques (BER). There are a number of systems under the general term of BER, such as the Mora and Indumed Therapy, Electro-acupuncture according to Voll (EAV) – which paved the way for the more successful VEGA test – and the Segmental Electrogram (SEG).

BER techniques are designed to register the bioelectrical potential at an acupuncture point. Because there is a direct relationship between acupuncture points and organs of the body, BER techniques are thus used to provide a diagnostic assessment of the organs, tissue systems and bodily functions corresponding to those points. The reasoning behind this is that when the body malfunctions, the electrical activity of the body is the first to be affected. This is followed by a chemical response and a pathological condition, or illness, may develop. BER testing is supposed to measure the electrical breakdown of the body before the chemical or pathological condition appears.

BER tests require no needles, are painless and are primarily used by naturopaths, homeopaths and acupuncturists because the information they provide is relevant to the holistic philosophy of diagnosing problems and treating them before disease or abnormal conditions actually appear.

VEGA Tests

VEGA tests use points on the skin to determine specific allergies. Vials of a possible allergic substance are transmitted through the Vega machine and the patient is connected to it. A probe is applied lightly to the "ting" points on the fingers and by measuring the responses of the patient the practitioner is supposed to be able to tell whether or not an allergy exists to the substance.

A Thera-tester operates on much the same principle as the VEGA machine. The EAV was the forerunner of the VEGA test but is a more cumbersome and complicated technique.

A number of practitioners in Australia are now using these techniques to test allergy responses.

Segmental electrogram (SEG)

The SEG machine records the body's energy reserves and its ability to react to a stimulus, detecting weakness or illness before the actual symptoms appear. The diagnosis involves placing electrodes at ten specific areas on the body. No sensation is felt but a mild stimulus is applied through the electrodes to obtain a computer readout.

Many asthma cases are chronic and asthma is often latent within the body; however, the SEG does not specifically tell if asthma is present, only if there is a deficiency or lower than usual reading in the segment that is being tested.

MIND OVER ASTHMA

Thought Patterns

If it is to be, it is up to me. These ten, two-letter words say so much. Repeat them. Think about them. They are easy to remember.

Worry, fear, anxiety and apprehension have a damaging effect on the glandular system and disrupt the body's natural harmony. Add poor nutrition and insufficient rest and you have the recipe for a depressed immune system. But a relaxed mind plus a relaxed body equals a positive healing response.

Changing your thought patterns from negative to positive, and setting achievable goals, are steps in the right direction towards physical and emotional wellness.

Start with simple goals, like going for a walk every day, doing Controlled Pattern Breathing exercises for 10 minutes when you wake up and eating a nutritious breakfast instead of skipping it. Small disciplines become habits and lead to major commitments. Goals and ambitions reflect your thoughts and if you think you can do something, like the Little Engine That Could, you will soon know you can.

You will be able to move on to bigger and better goals –
like aiming to lessen your asthma attacks by 50 per cent within
three months; or to play your favorite sport without relying on
an inhaler. Work on just one goal at a time but start now – today!
Write down your goal on a piece of paper and put it in a con-
spicuous place so you can read it every day. A copy on the
refrigerator door, your bathroom mirror and the dashboard of
your car will constantly remind you of your commitment and
reinforce your changed thought pattern.

Positive Thinking

Norman Vincent Peale, the author of *The Power of Positive*
Thinking, declares that all things are possible with positive
thoughts and attitudes. Countless books have been written ampli-
fying this theory. Similar philosophies, used by such renowned
authors as Dale Carnegie and more recently Louise L. Hay, teach
that our thoughts create our future.

Unhealthy thought patterns breed unhealthy bodies. Reversing negativity in our minds will reverse mental and physical conflict within our bodies. A positive desire is the starting point to
learning and adopting a positive attitude. The key to positive
changes is self acceptance and self approval. Feeling good about
ourselves gives us the confidence and determination to take
control of our lives and succeed in any endeavor.

Recovery from illness is impeded by anxiety, tension,
depression and nerves. The medical profession regularly sees the
outcome of positive and negative attitudes. People with happy
dispositions want to get better. They are up and out of bed in
no time. Their healing is faster and their recuperation time is less
than those who are unhappy, depressed or despondent. Instead
of being infected with disease you can become infected with
good health. Wanting to take charge of your asthma by taking
steps to improve your health is the reason you are reading this
book. Your positive attitude is already in place.

Consider the various ideas for turning your thinking around,
being positive wherever you have been negative in the past, then
try those that appeal to you. If you follow those that prove
helpful – starting with learning Controlled Pattern Breathing and

relaxation techniques – you are making a choice to be healthy.

One woman, Josie, who believed her asthma was due to her nervous tension and inferiority complex, was given the book *The Power from Within* (Spectrum Publications). The author, Elizabeth J. Cameron, had a severe physical disability but still had the same desires as everyone else. She asked: "Would I be able to have boyfriends, go to parties and dances? Would I ever marry, run a home, raise children? Would I be able to get enjoyment from life or would I just be a burden on society?" Are physical appearance, education, position, wealth or social upbringing the really important things in life? Her conclusion was that the most important factor in life is a person's mental outlook and his or her conduct and communication with other people. The book had such an impact on Josie that it prompted a dramatic change in her attitude to herself. She is now a much happier and more relaxed person and rarely has an attack of asthma.

So from now on do things you enjoy, that make you happy, make you laugh, make you feel good about yourself. No matter how old you are you can dwell on positive thoughts, imagine yourself in perfect health running happily along a beach or through a rain forest. You can listen to a running stream or water gurgling over rocks, the birds singing or your favorite music. Turn off the television, go for a walk, have a massage, talk to interesting people, meditate, go to church, practice a sport, get out in the garden, listen to relaxation tapes. Whether you are an asthmatic or have any other physical illness or handicap, a positive, healthy, happy attitude will help you make the most of your disability and ease its limitations. Conquering illness needs strength which can only come from the power within.

Autosuggestion

"My, you are looking well today!" "Hey, don't you look great today!" "Love your jacket, that color really suits you," "What have you been doing to look so healthy?," "I don't think I have seen you looking better" . . . the effect of comments like these is to put us on top of the world. A smile or kind, encouraging words from well-wishers cheer us when we are ill. And no one needs a smile more than the person who doesn't have one to give.

Compliments from **other** people fill us with pride and pleasure. If someone else can make us feel good by their words, isn't it feasible that **we** can do the same thing for **ourselves**?

Autosuggestion is simply complimenting and encouraging ourselves, to feel good within ourselves and to release the healing powers of mind and body – a sort of self-hypnosis. In recent decades, psychologists in our Western medical tradition have begun to realize just how much a patient's state of mind can influence his or her health.

Emile Coué (1857–1926), a French physician, developed the technique of autosuggestion and coined the now-famous phrase "Every day, in every way, I am getting better and better." Coué believed that a patient's will to live or get better was not enough if that patient had an imaginary fear of not recovering. Clearing the mind of all conscious thought, as in meditation, and regularly repeating his phrase activates the unconscious processes of the mind and body in a positive way.

In meditation we can listen to our inner thoughts and feelings or clear our minds of all distractions, and thus concentrate on healing our physical and emotional problems. Imagining and visualizing how we want to be or feel is reinforced by autosuggestion. Influencing the imagination by autosuggestion has become an integral part of many therapies to speed recovery and help relieve the pain and suffering of illnesses.

Autosuggestion can benefit everyone, but is particularly useful for anyone experiencing tension, anxiety, fear, asthma, allergy, psychosomatic illness and addictions to food, alcohol or smoking. It can be used to build your self-esteem, your confidence and your relationships. Just set aside some time night and morning to repeat – aloud or silently – one particular phrase or affirmation. You need to be completely relaxed and repeat your chosen phrase about 20 times, rather like an incantation.

Affirmations have to be worded positively and in the present tense: "I am" or "I have." The most renowned affirmations for pain or when recovering from illness are Coué's "Every day, in every way, I am getting better and better," and "I am totally healthy." For asthma or bronchitis you could say: "The breath of life flows easily through my body" or "I am asthma-free." If you are striving for relaxation and tranquillity try: "I am completely at peace" or "I am happy." To stop smoking, drinking or eating too much you could use: "I am a non-smoker," "Smoking is not good for my body, I have stopped smoking," "I am not eating chocolate today"or "I am not drinking alcohol – it harms my liver." For self-esteem: "I am independent and confident."

It is important that you phrase your affirmation positively and as attainable now. Negative statements like "I don't want to be fat" or "I don't want to be sick" dwell on what you don't want and will only create more of it. Using the future tense "I will" or "I want to" will keep your desires out of reach.

If you have difficulty mastering this self-help technique consult a qualified hypnotherapist or a clinical psychologist. Although psychotherapists can also help, always check their qualifications; they may only have limited training and so it may be unwise to rely on them.

AUTOSUGGESTION AND ASTHMA

Autosuggestion can turn negative perceptions into positive strengths for better health and happiness. It may be that your asthma responds to autosuggestion: you can only try it!

Hypnotherapy

Hypnotherapy is not suitable for children.

Primarily, hypnosis is an altered, trance-like state of mind or consciousness. Although the popular perception of someone under a hypnotic trance is like a sleepwalker, they are more often wide awake.

Hypnotherapy is used to bring about physical and mental changes to heal physical illness, reduce pain, induce relaxation or to recall past events. People in an hypnotic state remain in control and are able to exercise their own free will. They cannot be compelled to do anything contrary to their moral beliefs. However, while under hypnosis people think, act, behave and respond much more positively to suggestions, and suggestions can be left in their minds to influence future behavior.

Most people can be hypnotized within 4–5 minutes, provided they are cooperative and relaxed. In the early stages the therapist talks quietly to the patient, repeating suggestions that he is tired, or has the subject look at an object such as a spinning wheel. Eye muscles become tired, the eyelids become heavy and close involuntarily and the subject enters a light trance. At this stage simple movements can be performed on request, such as raising an arm. A deep hypnotic state follows and the patient becomes receptive to posthypnotic suggestions, or can be guided into past behavior.

When the mind and body are calmed and tranquil, or in a healing trance-like state, the ability to change becomes more accessible. A deep hypnotic state can also be used to eliminate any sense of pain, which is why surgery can be carried out on hypnotized patients without anesthetic.

The success of hypnotherapy is reflected in the fact that many medical practitioners have recognized its effectiveness in giving drug-free relief from pain and treating other problems, to the extent that they have become qualified hypnotherapists. Disorders that respond particularly well to hypnosis include stress and anxiety-related illnesses, skin disorders, migraine, irritable bowel syndrome, peptic ulcers, asthma and insomnia. Hypnosis can help overcome phobias and more common fears such as dislike of air travel, heights, exams or going to the dentist. Smoking, drug and alcohol addiction and eating disorders can be controlled with hypnosis.

The highest level of cooperation and trust must exist between the patient and the hypnotherapist. At the outset, therapists discuss the patient's problems, what they want to achieve, dispel any perceived concerns, and explain just what will happen during a session. Following 6–8 weekly sessions – or after an illness has been brought under control – most therapists teach their patients self-hypnosis. This is a very useful technique for people who need to use the power of suggestion at times when they are not in a consultation: insomniacs in the middle of the night; smokers reaching for a cigarette pack; or asthmatics worried they may be going to have an attack.

A word of warning: slick, entertaining hypnotists have put this therapy under suspicion, and too many worthless diplomas are being handed out after brief training courses. Associations of professional therapists exist all over the world and will verify qualifications, or will supply a list of appropriately qualified members. An unqualified hypnotherapist can implant damaging suggestions and do more harm than good, so always carefully check the credentials of any hypnotherapist you consult.

HYPNOTHERAPY AND ASTHMA

Hypnosis has been proved to be helpful for some asthmatics, especially those who panic when they realize they have come in contact with a trigger. Self-hypnosis is invaluable for people with asthma who need on-the-spot help. With self-hypnosis asthmatics can implant their own suggestions for breathing control to help their condition, and use the powers of hypnosis when they most need them: at the time an attack is imminent.

Meditation

Meditation allows the conscious mind to experience increasingly subtle states of thought until the source of the thought, the unlimited store of energy and creative intelligence, is reached. The mind settles effortlessly, thought dissolves altogether and a delicate state of silence is experienced.

The benefits of meditation come from expanding the mind's conscious capacity in order to remove deeply placed stresses from the body. Meditation dissolves everyday stresses and maintains a healthy, vibrant immune system.

The role of stress as the cause of illness has been as extensively researched as the role of meditation in reducing stress. The World Health Organization recently passed a resolution recommending meditation as a cost-effective health-care system. Major corporations find that meditation lifts the production levels of their staff, and sporting organizations that athletic performance is enhanced. High-powered business and professional people, politicians, office workers – in fact, people from all walks of life – have discovered the inner peace and outer health results from meditation. Instead of taking pain-relieving drugs, tranquillizers, sleeping pills and antidepressants, they are meditating. If everyone meditated, there would be much less need for expensive medical treatments.

Throughout India and Asia, meditation has been practiced for thousands of years. It wasn't until the late 1960s, when the Beatles and other pop musicians focused their attention on

Eastern music and culture, that masses of young people in the West adopted meditation in their search for alternative approaches to life's problems. The Maharishi Mahesh Yogi attracted many followers worldwide to his Transcendental Meditation, which requires chanting a secret, personal mantra – a phrase or sound. There are, however, numerous other systems and philosophies of meditation apart from the Maharishi's, which many people find preferable.

Meditating in a group does seem to be helpful for some: it frees them from interruptions and helps them stay focused and centred on their inward journey. They feel meditating in a group unifies people and creates strong healing vibrations to uplift mind, body and soul.

Meditation is easy to learn but does require concentration, persistence and time. Although group meditation or being taught is probably the simplest way to master the discipline, there are many books which will guide you thoroughly. We can only give a very brief description here.

HOW TO MEDITATE

Sit in a comfortable chair (or lie down) in a quiet room where you will not be interrupted. If sitting, rest your hands in your lap; if lying down have your arms by your side, palms up or facing towards your body. Your eyes can be open or closed but be wary of lying down with your eyes closed – you might just drop off to sleep.

The aim is to completely relax and stop unnecessary thoughts from entering your mind, clearing it to a calm state of nothingness. Initially, it is not easy to control thoughts, but focusing on just one thought stops others. That is why a mantra is sometimes used, as a meaningless phrase you can focus on. You can also focus on your breath – practice Controlled Pattern Breathing – concentrate on an object, or play a soothing tape to induce a meditative state. Guided meditation tapes are readily available from many alternative therapy outlets and stores.

MEDITATION AND ASTHMA

Stress is a known cause of asthma and meditation is a self-help way to ease stress, thus preventing asthma. The gentle breathing that is a part of meditation, and the reduced oxygen consumption that occurs when you are meditating, coupled with muscle relaxation, is just what asthma sufferers need to improve their condition. Meditating for 10–20 minutes a day can transform your life.

Yin and Yang, or Energy Balancing

A basis of Chinese philosophy is that in everything there are two opposing but complementary energy forces, which together make a balanced whole. Yin is a passive, protecting force and yang a positive, driving force. Yin patterns are equated with the interior, deficiency and cold, whereas yang is associated with the exterior, excess and heat. The sun, for instance, is classified as yang and the moon as yin; day as yang and night as yin. Broadly speaking, the concept of yang and yin is hot/cold, sun/moon, male/female, day/night, health/sickness, summer/winter, white/black, spring/autumn, above the ground/under the ground, full/empty, acid/alkaline.

As the yin/yang symbol illustrates, there is always some yin within yang and some yang within yin. For example, although midnight is completely yin and midday completely yang, twilight and early morning are both yin and yang. There are some male characteristics within a female and some female characteristics in a male, but male is described as yang and female as yin. Yin constantly moves towards yang and yang towards yin to maintain harmony and balance.

Confusing, you may think? Well, not in Chinese philosophy and medicine. Health, the Chinese believe, is the result of a balance of yin and yang within the body. An imbalance leads to illness. Internal illnesses are believed to stem from too much yin, whereas problems caused by external agents such as climate, infection and allergy are the effect of excess yang. Rather than focusing on symptoms, Chinese medicine uses acupressure, acupuncture, moxibustion, shiatsu, reflexology and t'ai-chi to stimulate the *chi* energy flow and build up whichever of the two forces is deficient.

According to this philosophy, whether we are resting or on the move, asleep or awake, hot or cold, the body is constantly in the process of energy balancing. When we get a fever, yin and yang disharmony can cause asthma, bronchitis, sinusitis, hay fever and other illnesses. Perhaps confusingly to Western thought, chronic asthma is said to come from a yin deficiency, whereas yang may be deficient when asthma is acute.

Diagnosis is based on a combination of yin and yang patterns and how the symptoms relate to a person's entire body and behavior pattern. Treatment is then recommended to balance the disharmony of the body's yin and yang.

YIN AND YANG AND ASTHMA

There are similarities between yin and yang and the philosophy behind Ron's treatment of asthma. It is Ron's belief that asthma can be relieved by counterbalancing what happens during an attack. For instance, the asthmatic's very short breathing pattern is balanced by the long breaths of the Controlled Pattern Breathing.

Color Therapy

Color affects us in many ways. It can change our mood, make us feel confident, increase our ability to concentrate, enhance our physical and mental aptitude and attitude, uplift us or help us recover from illness. Yes, it really can! Increasing scientific evidence about the body's responses to colors has led to specific colors being used in mental health clinics, hospital recovery rooms, prison cells, workplaces and to stimulate retarded children.

Our subtle senses react to bright colors – they enliven us – whereas dull colors seem to dampen our enthusiasm. Color is also a significant factor in the marketing and advertising of products to tempt consumers to buy. Psychologists are consulted by large corporations to assess prospective employees by testing their color preferences. How does it work? Color in lights, food and surroundings is believed to stimulate the nervous system to increase hormone production, thus affecting the body's chemical and energy balance.

Color therapy is as old as the Healing Temples of Light and Color which stood at Heliopolis in ancient Egypt. It has been used for thousands of years by the Chinese. In our culture, recent extensive American experiments into color for health revealed that when people were "bathed" in blue light their blood pressure dropped significantly, but being "bathed" in red light speeded up circulation and caused blood pressure to rise.

An English researcher, Theo Gimbel, found blue to be the healing, calming color and of most benefit in treating an asthma attack. Emerald green was most favorable for hay fever, influenza, colds, ulcers and malaria. Orange appeared to activate the respiratory system. Gimbel also researched the link between visualization of color and diet, using foods of specific colors. His experiments showed visualizing orange and eating orange-colored fruit or vegetables were most favorable for asthma sufferers and for coughs, colds and bronchitis.

Some color therapists believe that various electromagnetic components of light are absorbed by the body which then emits its own aura of colors. An unbalanced pattern of aura vibrations indicates an unhealthy body.

Color therapy may not be as widely practiced as other complementary healing modalities, but many therapists offer it as another way to promote physical well-being and emotional uplifting. According to many therapists color therapy treatment has helped asthma, migraine, eczema, insomnia, stress, high blood pressure, lack of energy and depression.

COLOR THERAPY AND ASTHMA

Experimenting with color can be a lot of fun. Think about what different colors do for you and surround yourself with those that make you feel good. Repaint your bedroom, put some bright new cushions on your chairs, throw out those drab colored clothes, be outlandish and buy yourself a happy colored dress, sweater, shirt, tie or socks. Glow in a kaleidoscope of color. What have you got to lose? Of course, make sure they are the right colors for you. Try blues, greens and orange. Gimbel says people with asthma should avoid red and black.

Maybe something as simple as a color change will make you feel great, then you'll look terrific and, when someone compliments you, your self-esteem will soar. It just may be the lift you need.

Spiritual Healing

More things are wrought by prayer than this world dreams of . . .
    – "The Idylls of the King," Alfred, Lord Tennyson

Spiritual healing and miracle cures have always baffled the calculating, rational world of scientists and medicine. But there is no denying it: countless cures have been attributed to a force that cannot be measured or explained by medical science.

The ancient tradition of faith or spiritual healing has been embraced by many different religions, and in modern times has been associated with Christianity. Most churches have some form of healing ritual, whether it be simple prayers for the sick at weekly services or special individual bedside services. Religious systems such as Christian Science preach spiritual healing as part of their creed.

The vast numbers of visitors to shrines famed for miracle cures, such as Lourdes in France, reflect the powerful Christian belief in Jesus's preaching of "thy faith hath made thee whole" and the efficacy of prayer. Disciples of St. Paul, a fervent believer in the Holy Spirit, prompted the evolution from more traditional churches of Pentecostal, Charismatic and Revivalist denominations, with their emphasis on the power of faith. Such charismatic groups hold prayer meetings and services to deliver healing.

The power of faith and prayer cannot be underestimated. Faith can move mountains. "Right" thinking, or the power within, puts the potential to heal within the reach of us all.

Discovering the power of faith and prayer has changed the lives of many people. Diseases have been cured or gone into remission, illnesses overcome and deformities corrected. Many people with asthma will verify that their faith and prayer have been a comfort to them and given them the strength to cope with their distressing condition. Others affirm that they have gained relief from faith healers and are grateful to such people who have developed and use their skill to perform acts of healing.

Faith healers rely on a person's belief, and work on the principle that whatever one believes can be made to happen. Extending someone's consciousness to be "in tune" with a higher level of spirituality, with God, a Supreme Being or whatever the "force" is conceived to be, opens remarkable possibilities for cure.

The orthodox medical profession theorizes that faith healers simply reinforce the mental attitudes of patients and they feel better, even if their actual condition is not cured. The body's natural defenses actively respond to the belief, stress is reduced, health-giving hormones may be produced and antibodies – the cells in the blood that fight infection and disease – are strengthened.

Ron's decision to stop smoking was the result of a healing service he attended 20 years ago. Smoking up to 30 cigarettes a day was not an easy addiction to overcome, but it was one of the most significant decisions of his life.

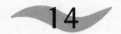

SOME ESOTERIC THERAPIES AND TECHNIQUES

Following is a brief overview of other esoteric therapies whose features may appeal to you and which you might like to explore further on your voyage of self discovery. Some of these therapies are not widely accessible but you will probably be able to obtain more comprehensive information about them from your local community center, library, complementary practitioner or health food store. We cannot recommend any of them as proven ways to improve asthma, but if they appeal to you they may do some good.

ART THERAPY
Painting, drawing or sketching are relaxing hobbies if done in an unpressured environment of not having to perform or "get it right." They inspire self expression, put many people in touch with thoughts and feelings they weren't aware of and release tension and frustration for many.

AURA SOMA
This combines the healing properties of colors, aromatherapy, plant extracts and crystal energies. It uses a range of 94 dual-

colored "balance bottles." Developed by Vicky Wall, an English apothecary and chiropodist, Aura Soma relies on the self-selection of balance bottle colors you are particularly drawn to. The meaning of the colors is supposed to enhance self-knowledge of your life's purpose and balance your life on all levels: spiritual, mental, emotional and physical. The chosen balance bottle liquid is applied to your body by self-massage.

BIOENERGETICS
Negative attitudes and emotions such as fear, anger, personal psychological problems and stress are expressed in the way we sit, stand, move and breathe. Bioenergetics makes us aware of poor habitual postures and body movements and uses exercises to unlock this "character armoring" and the associated emotions. The body thus regains its ability to function freely producing a more positive attitude, for improved energy and vitality.

Bioenergetics concentrates on personal growth rather than curing illness, although help has been reported with migraine, asthma, irritable bowel syndrome and peptic ulcers.

BIOFEEDBACK
In biofeedback, machines monitor changes in physical and mental states and provide information so that the patient can control body functions using such techniques as breathing and relaxation, meditation and visualization therapy. Although many of the internal workings of our body are not under our conscious control, through biofeedback it is possible to learn to influence them. Thus blood pressure, skin temperature, digestion and muscular tension can all be controlled. Whether asthma can be helped using biofeedback is unclear, but it has certainly been proved that blood pressure can be reduced without taking drugs by using biofeedback machines.

BIORHYTHMS
Three internal body clocks or cycles are thought to control physical, emotional and intellectual ups and downs. It is believed that by understanding the relationship between the pattern of biorhythms and our pattern of behavior we can chart our lives, thus being able to recognize difficult days and make the most of favorable days.

COLONIC IRRIGATION

Cleansing the body of "impurities" is often suggested by naturopaths to give it a rest from the constant assault of toxic matter. Colonic irrigation and enemas are frequently recommended to treat chronic constipation, biliousness or indigestion, conditions often associated with asthma, as well as for general cleansing. Colonic irrigation and enemas should only be carried out in a sterile environment by qualified practitioners and with a physician's approval. Although colonic irrigation may seem a rather drastic measure to treat asthma, and one unconnected with breathing, it is possible that ridding the body of toxic and waste matter improves health and well-being generally.

CRYSTAL THERAPY

Naturally-occurring crystals, including precious and semiprecious stones, are said to contain positive energy which strengthens other treatments. Crystals are either placed on the body parts which need help, on particular acupuncture points or can be worn or carried close to the body. Rose quartz is used for emotional healing, quartz for physical healing and amethyst for spiritual healing.

DANCE MOVEMENT THERAPY

Flowing, graceful, uninhibited, letting-go movements to music relax the mind and body, ease tension and release pent-up emotions. Try doing this on a warm day, in an open parkland, with no shoes on and eyes closed (if you can). Even without music the feeling of freedom is delightful.

DO-IN

This ancient form of Chinese self-massage in the form of a series of exercises is aimed at preventing rather than curing disease, by strengthening energy channels linked to the heart, lungs, liver, gallbladder and other organs. Do-in is related to shiatsu and some of the exercises and positions are similar to yoga postures.

GESTALT OR HUMANISTIC PSYCHOLOGY

This promotes personal growth by self-awareness, resolving inner conflict and taking control of one's ideas, actions and feelings to release anxiety and tension and restore emotional self-confidence.

HELLERWORK

Concentrates on the connective fascia tissue that wraps around the bundles of fibers making up muscles. It works on mind–body integration in a way similar to rolfing and the Alexander technique, restoring balance to the body, relaxing and releasing accumulated stress and tension.

IRIDOLOGY

Iridologists believe that markings and changes in the irises of the eyes can locate and diagnose mind and body problems. Experienced iridologists are capable of recognizing early warning signs of illnesses before symptoms arise and recommend patients see their doctor. Iridology is often liked by people who are uneasy with the blood tests, X-rays, swabs and biopsies of conventional medicine.

MACROBIOTICS

A diet of vegetables and whole grains based on using a balance of yin and yang foods to complement the yin and yang in a person's condition (see page 192–3).

MUSIC AND SOUND THERAPY

Organs and cells in the body are thought by followers of this therapy to have natural resonance, and to respond well to sounds that vibrate in harmony with it. Thus vibrations and rhythmic breathing can alter electrical brain wave patterns.

The frequency of cell and organ vibrations is affected by poor health and disease. Dissonant sounds from noisy equipment, low flying jets, rush-hour traffic are irritating and create anxiety and tension, while harmonious rhythms ease pent-up emotions, which can cause distressing emotional and physical problems.

The power of sound is reflected in how theme songs excite and unify sporting fans and why piped music is used in shopping centers to lull people into staying longer and spending more. Listening to pleasant music is a great way to unwind after a stressful day and "new age" music composed with distinctive harmonious vibrations is even more calming and relaxing.

POLARITY BALANCING

Polarity balancing uses the natural currents of life-force that flow through everyone's hands to release the blockages in the body's energy currents that cause symptoms of illness. When the currents flow naturally illness can be overcome, balance and health restored. Therapy involves manipulation and touch, stretching postures, diet and positive mental attitude.

PYRAMID POWER

Theories that pyramid shapes create heightened energy fields, which can alter the rate of physical, chemical and biological processes that take place inside them, are still being researched. Brain activity patterns of people have been found to change noticeably inside pyramids and the subjects reported feeling "warm, tingling sensations." Pyramid power is believed to increase vitality, relieve toothache, headaches, cramps, rheumatic pain and tension, prompt sounder sleep and improve well-being.

REICHIAN THERAPY

Not to be confused with reiki, Reichian therapy (which is also known as orgone therapy) focuses on how posture, muscular tension – called body armoring by Reichians – and breathing patterns reflect emotions. Physical manipulation, it is believed, relaxes body armoring and releases muscle tension, thus freeing repressed emotions.

The leader of the movement, psychiatrist William Reich, was born in Austria in 1897 and graduated as an M.D. in 1922. He worked closely with Sigmund Freud for a short while but, like many others at this time, had differences of opinion with Freud and they parted company. Reich moved to America in 1939 and accepted a post in medical psychology in New York. Reich wrote numerous books and believed strongly in the concept of bio-energy flow through the body. He considered that repression of the emotions and sexual instincts could lead to "orgone energy" blockages, resulting in rigid patterns of behavior and tightening of specific muscle groups. This, he believed, led to a marked deterioration of health.

Reich devised an "orgone accumulator," a box made of metal

and wood in layers in which he could "concentrate" orgone like an electrical charge. Patients sat in the box, supposedly to have this energy restored.

In 1950 an experiment went horribly wrong. A reaction occurred between orgone and the radium he was using while trying to demonstrate that orgone could counteract the dangers of radiation. All the Orgone Institute's mice died and many workers were affected by radiation sickness. Much adverse publicity followed Reich through a number of years of other orgone energy experiments, which finally led to his arrest. American government authorities ordered all his accumulators, equipment and printed matter destroyed on the basis that orgone energy did not exist. Reich died in jail of a heart attack in 1957.

Although Reich's theories have been rejected by many psychologists and scientists, some of his ideas and methods are still considered credible and have undergone a recent revival. It would appear, though, that with only a small number of followers and a lack of evidence on which to assess Reich's theories there are few practicing therapists.

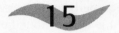

LIFESTYLE APPROACHES

Coping with Stress

Stress is a major trigger of asthma. All of us experience stress every day of our lives. How we respond to it and cope with it is reflected in our state of health. Changes in our lives, new and constant demands on our time and our attention, instant decisions to be made, are all stressful. Stress is individual, though: we give it to ourselves, which is why some people are more upset than others by the same event.

Don't forget that stress can be good – challenges and changes can fire our enthusiasm, spur us on to greater achievements, add excitement to our lives; this is positive stress. Stress is only dangerous when we fail to adapt to pressures and problems and our reactions create feelings of frustration, anxiety, anger, impatience and anguish – negative stress.

Balanced stress is the key to a happy and healthy body. We can avoid stress by eliminating its causes – not driving in traffic, quitting the job, putting the crying child in another room, taking the phone off the hook. But when we cannot avoid stress we worry. We worry about paying bills, work pressures, exams, family arguments . . . or having another attack of asthma.

Avoiding problems or worrying about them does not help

us handle them any better. The secret of balanced stress is learning to cope with the underlying causes. Even though we may
not have control over the events around us, we can have control
over how we react to them and minimize their effects.

To create a balanced life, one that flows easily rather than
one that is a struggle, we must first want to have a balanced
mind and body. An important part of being out of balance is
that often we don't feel like doing anything about it. But you
have to make the effort, for releasing yourself from unnecessary
stress will release your body from the burden of asthma.

There is no single path to a more balanced, less stressed life.
This book continually emphasizes the importance of relaxation
and contains a selection of enjoyable techniques for you to try.
Start today – take the following steps.

1 Identify the causes of stress in your life. Draw up a list
  of what is currently stressing you, including the good
  things – for instance, a new baby brings joy but also
  sleepless nights, disrupted domestic routine and strained
  family relationships.
2 Consider your reactions. Do you meet a problem head
  on, even before it occurs? Your aggression is showing
  and you are putting yourself at risk from heart
  disorders. Are you fixed in your ways and attitude and
  object to changes in your life? Such inflexibility can
  create digestive disorders such as irritable bowel
  syndrome and stomach ulcers. Do you avoid problems,
  pretend they don't exist or leave them to other people?
  Relinquishing control, becoming dependent on others,
  leads to withdrawal and, some practitioners believe,
  increases the risk of developing cancer.
3 Vary your reactions. If you are responding the same
  way all the time to every problem you are not
  responding appropriately. Think about the alternative
  ways you can react.
4 Maintain stress awareness. Now you know you can
  control your reactions, take time out at night and
  reflect on your responses to the day's events. Review
  the possibilities and alternatives for the day ahead.
5 Be self nurturing. Look after yourself with a healthy

diet, exercise regularly, get a good night's sleep, practice breathing techniques, meditate, take up yoga or t'ai-chi and pamper yourself with some of the many relaxing therapies suggested in this book. Laugh a lot.

There is no doubt that asthma has a stress-related factor. The stress doesn't have to come from outside, though. Asthma tends to be more common during puberty, menstruation, pregnancy and change of life: situations you can't avoid. So the body is not only under duress at these times but also has to work hard to counteract the asthma.

When our bodies suffer physical pain or the discomfort of asthma, our immune system has to work overtime. It, too, becomes stressed as it strives to function efficiently. The stress increases, and it can become a vicious circle. What is the answer? Take a vacation? Sure, great idea, but it will reduce the bank balance and probably lead to even more stresses . . . And so the stress carousel keeps turning.

Fundamentally, you have two choices. Relieve the physical problem – such as asthma – first and you will relieve one of the major stresses in your life, or reduce your stress and minimize the likelihood of asthma and other stress-related illnesses. Whichever you choose, your goal is to achieve a life filled with only positive stress and physical and emotional balance.

Allergies

What allergies are and how they cause asthma was described in detail in Part One of this book. This section is focusing on how to prevent allergies causing asthma by lifestyle approaches.

Often it isn't just the allergy itself that is the problem, though. Most asthmatics have a poor medical history and their usually depleted immune system lowers their resistance to diseases in general, and makes them more susceptible to invasions from allergens. Add to this scenario poor diet, hormonal imbalance and stress, and you may find trying to conquer ill health becomes a constant battle. All the stress of fighting asthma can increase the frequency and severity of allergic reactions.

Every asthmatic has individual triggers which he needs to

clearly identify so they can be eliminated, treated or, at least, avoided. You can track down your own allergies by simply keeping a diary of how substances, environments or activities influence your asthma. Most trigger factors will cause symptoms almost immediately – within 30 minutes or so. You might, for instance, start to wheeze shortly after vacuuming the house, gardening, exercising, wearing a particular perfume or drinking a glass of wine. If you are sensitive to foods your observations may reveal a pattern linked to additives. Confirmation of your allergic sensitivities can be carried out by your doctor using skin prick tests or scratch tests. RAST (radioallergosorbent) tests, a type of blood test, are also used in some cases.

Here are some precautions you can take to minimize allergic asthma.

- Check your diet – eat preservative-, chemical- and additive-free foods.
- Use allergen-proof bedding. All sheets, pillows and blankets should be of a natural material; avoid polyester as your body warmth will release its hydrocarbons, which may cause problems. Vacuum mattresses frequently and don't store anything under your bed.
- An electric blanket has positive and negative factors. If you are allergic to dust mites you can keep their population down in your bedding by turning on an electric blanket to full power for a couple of hours a week. Do it during the day, when you aren't in bed. This won't kill the mites, but it will dry the bedding out, which mites don't like.

    However, you should **not** use an electric blanket when you are in the bed. It might keep you cozy, but its wires are sealed in plastic and when heated give off an invisible vapor that asthmatics do better to avoid.
- Avoid wall-to-wall carpets and loose furnishings that cannot be easily washed at high temperatures. Have polished floors and scatter rugs.
- Steam-cleaning won't kill mites: the temperature isn't hot enough and all it does is make the environment the mite lives in more humid and warmer – exactly the conditions it thrives in!

- Make sure your house is well ventilated.
- Indoor plants contribute oxygen to your home, but don't keep too many as wet dirt causes molds and fungi to grow, which release spores that may be an allergen.
- Don't keep a pet if you are allergic to it. If you can't give up the family pet try to ensure it lives outside.
- Keep your living and working areas dry and clothes well aired and free of any dampness.
- Keep bathrooms well ventilated to prevent mold.
- Dry clothing and bedding inside, or in a dryer, instead of outside where they can pick up pollen.
- Plant a garden with minimal wind-pollinated plants. Use paving or gravel instead of lawn.
- Create a pollutant-free haven or sanctuary in one room of the house – perhaps your bedroom. You can then escape to this room during an attack.

All these suggestions are ways to avoid triggers in your life, but you can go much further. It is possible to design a house that minimizes exposure to a wide range of triggers. The Asthma Foundation of Victoria, Australia, has produced plans for a Breathe-Easy house, with electric heating and cooking appliances, special insulation and ventilation systems, easy-to-clean surfaces, low-allergy paint, and so on. There are also environmentally friendly builders in the U.S. and U.K.

Environmental Pollution

Pollution is the price the world has had to pay for progress. Before the Industrial Revolution pollution was virtually unknown except for the natural phenomena of volcanic eruptions, swamps emitting methane gas, sulphur springs or fires. Industrialization has exposed us to an enormous amount of man-made irritants. The human body is now forced to cope with constant health hazards in the form of water and air pollution, noise, stress, radiation and dangerous chemicals, forced upon us from factories, power stations, agriculture, mines and waste disposal.

Environmental pollution has brought about an alarming

increase in respiratory diseases and this alone may well be the major cause of today's high incidence of asthma, particularly in industrial areas. Although not attacked with such a vengeance, nonurban areas are not without hazards, with air and water pollution from agricultural pesticides and burn-offs. Most people with asthma will recognize car exhaust fumes as a trigger, but it is not generally recognized that aircraft burn enormous amounts of fuel, and their exhaust is spread throughout the atmosphere. People who live near airports may be breathing enough aircraft pollution for this to be a significant asthma trigger.

Pollutants from fertilizers, pesticides, detergent washing powders and industrial wastes foul rivers, lakes, reservoirs and our domestic water. Then chemicals such as chlorine, fluoride and aluminum are added to our water supplies to complete the health-destroying cocktail.

Fruit and vegetables are grown with artificial fertilizers and sprayed with chemicals. Animals are treated with artificial hormones to increase their weight, with antibiotics to prevent disease and are reared on crops sprayed with chemicals. Food additives, preservatives and artificial flavorings and colorings, combined with plastic wrapping and packaging, adulterate our food. Then we chew all this polluted food with amalgam-filled teeth which add excess mercury to our slowly poisoning bodies.

And we don't just have to worry about outside pollution. Inside, our homes and workplaces are riddled with pollutants. Gas stoves and heaters emit nitrogen dioxide, aging refrigeration still contains chlorofluorocarbons (CFCs), radiation comes from television screens, microwave ovens, fluorescent lamps and computers. Insulating materials, paints, carpets, glues, tobacco smoke, ovens, vacuum cleaners, air conditioning, all emit fumes, irritants or radiation, and the list goes on.

In the last thirty years we have become surrounded by electromagnetic fields, not just from household appliances but also from living near high-tension power lines. When we have something wrong with us we are X-rayed, and now scientists talk of X-raying our food! We are trapped in a radiation filled world.

Millions of office workers spend most of their waking lives in artificially controlled atmospheres that are potentially hazardous to their health. Severe illnesses such as allergic reactions, hay fever, asthma attacks and repeated respiratory infections plague employees of badly ventilated offices, and absenteeism impairs productivity for the employer and industry in general. In many situations, the major culprit is inefficient air conditioning. Poorly planned installations do not allow effective access to areas that need to be kept clean and dry to prevent them becoming a breeding ground for fungi and bacteria. Often the air is contaminated due to badly situated intakes being affected by car emissions from the parking lot or garage. Some buildings have practically no fresh air intake at all, as building managers wanting to save running costs recirculate too much air because they believe it is cheaper than having to heat or cool fresh air.

There is undeniable evidence that the environment can make us ill. Headaches, fatigue, insomnia, eye disorders, irritation of the throat, lungs and respiratory tract, asthma, allergy, emphysema, bronchitis, immune system damage, memory loss, cancer and defects in newborn babies can be traced to pollution. There is evidence that 20 per cent of hospital admissions of people with asthma attacks were the result of environmental pollution.

And the environmental pollutants **continue** to increase asthma in our society. However, if you believe that pollution is the major contributing factor to your asthma there is much you can do to make your environment healthier. You can take control of your condition and reduce or eliminate your exposure to household and workplace pollutants.

- Keep everything that gives off unpleasant odors out of inhalation range until you need to use them. These include polishes, window and oven cleaners, insecticides, cosmetics, nail polish and remover, glues, etc. Use only in well-ventilated areas.
- Don't buy expensive aerosol cleaners; make your own with natural ingredients.
- Disconnect your automatic gas stove pilot light – a constant source of gas seepage – and keep gas use to a minimum. In just one hour cooking at 180°C (350°F) a gas oven emits enough carbon monoxide and nitrogen dioxide fumes to trigger an allergic attack.
- Use lead-free paint and gasoline.
- Wash your clothes (and your dishes) in detergent-free biodegradable washing soda or soap. Chemicals in

washing powders cling to garments and then penetrate your skin.

- Buy clothes made from natural fibers like cotton or wool, not synthetics.
- Choose cosmetics, perfumes, soaps and hair products made from plant extracts rather than mineral oils.
- Use an electric razor and ordinary ice water as an astringent.
- Wherever possible choose unpackaged foods or products in glass. Plastic food wrappings leach out pollutants and contaminate food. Avoid plastic cookware and servingware, too.
- Limit alcoholic intake as it can cause swelling of blood vessels in the nasal passages.
- Don't smoke, and stay out of smoke-filled rooms. Fireplaces, wood stoves and cigarettes are fuel for asthma.
- Ensure your heating and cooling systems, and exhaust fans in your home and car, work efficiently.
- Rid your garden of pests with herbs, not insecticides.
- Sit at least two meters away from the television.
- Polyurethane foam, found in seat cushions, food and other packaging, and refrigerator insulation, contains the chemical isocyanate, which is believed to have led to a dramatic increase in respiratory ailments such as asthma. Avoid where at all possible.
- Move to a less polluted area or climate if possible.

ALTERNATE NOSTRIL BREATHING

Your nose, the body's air-conditioner, can clear accumulated allergens, pollutants and irritants which clog your nasal cavities and respiratory tract, to give speedy relief from asthma attacks, dust sensitivities and stubborn coughs. Five minutes a day of alternate nostril breathing will clean out irritants, help you breathe better and strengthen your immunity to allergies.

> ▶ Place your index finger on your forehead between your
>   eyebrows, with thumb on one side of your nose and
>   bent middle finger on the other.
> ▶ Breathe in through both nostrils. Close one nostril with
>   your finger and breathe out via the other side.
> ▶ Breathe in through this same side, close, and release
>   closed nostril, breathe out.
> ▶ Breathe in through same side, close, release closed
>   nostril and breathe out.
> ▶ This is "one round" – repeat a minimum of four times
>   at least once or twice each day.

If one side of your nose is blocked, breathe in through the clear
nostril, close and breathe out through the other. If both nostrils
are blocked, breathe in through your mouth and forcibly out
through alternate nostrils until one or other – or both – clear,
and you can stop the mouth breathing.

Smoking

Quit now!

Even representatives of the tobacco industry agree that it is sensible for people with asthma to avoid cigarette smoke. Legislation
has enforced smoking restrictions in public buildings around the
world. Exposure to cigarette smoke, even while in the womb,
and particularly during the first year of life is likely to increase
a child's risk of developing asthma. Years of exposure to cigarette
smoke can result in irreversible lung damage and for an asthmatic
the problem can be exacerbated.

In November 1993, the *Journal of the American Medical
Association* singled out tobacco as the number one culprit in
causing death in the U.S. Heart disease and cancer were listed
as the nation's leading killers, but the underlying cause of death
was the use of tobacco. The research found that smoking contributed to the deaths of 400,000 Americans in 1990 – more than
those caused by drug use, guns and car accidents put together.

Rating second to tobacco came poor diet and lack of exercise.

Asthma sufferers often say that smoking helps relieve their asthma and that's why they don't want to give it up. Yes, in the short term smoking can relieve asthma. Why? Because smoking helps people relax – the nicotine in the cigarette can relax the bronchi – and smokers breathe in short and breathe out long and slow. Sounds familiar? Of course, for these are the two major concepts of asthma relief contained in this book – relaxation and controlled breathing. But smoking will also *produce* asthma in the medium term and leads to cancer and emphysema.

Just one cigarette lowers lung capacity, narrows the arteries, raises blood pressure, tenses the muscles and puts extra strain on the heart for an hour and a half after you have smoked it. Tobacco also depletes Vitamin B1, Vitamin B3, Vitamin B6, Vitamin C, magnesium and zinc stores in the body, which saps your vitality, makes you lethargic and prone to infection.

If you are a parent there is added incentive to give up smoking. There is substantial evidence that children who grow up in homes where cigarette smoke is present have increased frequency of asthma. Dr Des Mulcahey, a pediatrician, has stated that a disproportionate number of parents of children admitted to the hospital with asthma attacks are heavy smokers. Studies indicate that passive smoking increases the risk of an asthma attack by approximately 50 per cent.

Children's lungs are ultrasensitive and when constantly exposed to smoke they are more likely to suffer from coughs, bronchitis and respiratory problems, including asthma and pneumonia, and have a greater risk of developing lung cancer. It has been argued that if smoking in the home was stopped, as many as one-third of asthmatic children would be helped.

If you are a smoker, consider what you are doing to your body – wrecking it. You are also wrecking your children's health, and that of people around you. Having read this book you now know you can improve your asthma using the many techniques and suggestions we have given you. Look after your body and it will look after you.

Sometimes you need to analyze why you are smoking to be able to stop.

●   Do you find yourself holding a cigarette that you can't

remember lighting? If you don't even know that you are having the cigarette, why have it at all!

- Do you smoke to calm down or to help you concentrate under pressure? There are far better ways to handle stress that won't harm your health like smoking does. Try exercise, meditation or relaxation.

- Do you smoke when you are feeling bad, to help you feel better? Smoking is only an instant fix. There are much more enjoyable ways you can feel better **all the time**. Work out a reward system for when you need a lift, and give yourself a present instead of a cigarette.

- Do you think you smoke a cigarette purely for the pleasure of it? Perhaps you believe this as a way of denying your addiction. Face up to it. Consider this: where's the pleasure in paying money to smell disgusting, ruin your health and alienate your friends?

- Do you smoke when you are absorbed in a particular project or pastime? If you don't, it's because your mind is totally occupied, which tells you that your mind can control your desire to smoke.

- Do you feel an urge to smoke when you see other people smoking? Peer group pressure is controlling and intimidating you. Be an individual.

- Do you find it hard to refuse an offer of a cigarette? Your willpower has deserted you; be determined and find it again.

- Do you usually have a cigarette first thing in the morning? Do diaphragmatic breathing exercises instead – they're much better for you.

- Do you crave a cigarette if you haven't had one for a couple of hours? If you can go this long, kick the addiction, don't pick up a cigarette – have an apple instead.

Stopping

What are you going to do about stopping? Make the decision right now, and **Quit**. Resist the temptation to have that last cigarette. Throw away the pack (and the lighter), put the ashtrays away in a cupboard. Tell everyone you have stopped smoking, and seek the support of your family, your friends and your workmates.

If you need help, there are courses for those trying to quit. Check the phone book, your local community center or doctor's office: you should be able to find a local group nearby you can join. Arm yourself with chewing gum (nicotine or otherwise) and barley sugar. If you need to you can use nicotine patches to help you over the first days or weeks. Increase your consumption of Vitamin C. Try homeopathic remedies to ease your addiction: these are easily obtainable at health food stores or pharmacies.

Enjoy the financial incentive. Just work out how much you used to spend on cigarettes each week (most people are horrified when they do). How much is that a year? That would pay for a terrific vacation, even a new car over a couple of years. Save the money you used to spend on cigarettes and give yourself a special treat. At least once a week reward yourself by buying or doing something that makes **you** feel good.

Hypnotherapy and acupuncture are extremely successful treatments for cigarette addictions. Try autosuggestion to reinforce your decision and help you overcome the subconscious desire to smoke. Buy tape recordings with stop smoking messages and play them repeatedly. Keep photographs nearby of lung damage caused by smoking.

Here are some tips to help in difficult times.

- Keep clearly in your mind why you smoked and why you have stopped.
- Avoid situations where the urge to smoke is strong.
- Confront the problem straight on.
- Change your routine.
- Go for an early morning walk.
- Vary the places where you usually sit.
- Put positive notes on the mirror or refrigerator.
- Exercise during a work break.
- Chew gum or suck lollipops and sweets (in moderation).
- Have a glass of water beside you all the time.
- Keep busy doodling or writing when you are on the phone.
- Remove the ashtrays and cigarette lighter from the car as well as the house.

- Whenever possible avoid being with people who smoke.
- Tell your friends you have stopped.
- Condition yourself to say: "No thanks, I have stopped smoking."
- Brush your teeth more frequently.
- Use a mouthwash after meals to freshen your mouth.
- Only go to nonsmoking restaurants.
- Take Vitamin C tablets.
- Actually plan the dream vacation you are going to have with the money saved. Book it as soon as you can. If the vacation becomes real it's an added incentive.

Stand firm on your decision to stop smoking, be confident with your conviction and your strength will be rewarded. Quit today – **you can do it!**

Weather

Climate and weather can enliven and invigorate us, or plunge us into bleak moods and low spirits. Fresh mountain air, a warm sunny day – and we are off outside, going for a walk, enjoying ourselves and we feel great. Gray skies, it's cold and raining – we stay inside, in overheated and often poorly ventilated homes and buildings, we don't exercise and really can't be bothered.

People with super-sensitive airways are more vulnerable to even the smallest fluctuation in weather conditions. Although scientists are not certain why, humidity and temperature changes do have a marked effect on asthma. Some asthmatics are upset by hot, dry weather and summer thunderstorms, others by cold damp airstreams, autumn mists or fog. Even indoor temperature changes can intensify an attack.

Unfortunately there isn't a lot we can do about weather. We certainly can't avoid it! However, if you know what your asthma trigger is you are more likely to be able to take precautions to minimize exposure to it. If you are sensitive to pollens then avoid wind, or going out just after rain when the pollen granules may have burst. If sudden heat or cold bring on asthma don't enter greenhouses or ice rinks.

Allergens blow through open windows of our homes and

mix with those already there. By air conditioning your house you can alleviate trigger problems. Air conditioning units keep humidity low, which discourages mites and molds, and in the course of cooling it will also filter the air if you install an air cleaner. In effect you can turn your home into an allergen-free sanctuary by sealing the house, instead of having the windows open to incoming pollens. Likewise, air condition your car but run it on the recirculate setting, not on the setting that pulls in outside air and cools it – cool, pollinated air is bad for asthma. But remember that unless you keep air conditioners, humidifiers and air filters scrupulously clean you may end up blowing allergens all round your home instead of eliminating them. Clean and wash appliance filters once a month.

With some planning you can do much to tame allergies caused by the weather.

- Stay indoors when pollen levels are highest – between 4 a.m. and 10 a.m.
- Buy a big scarf to keep your mouth and nose covered when you are outdoors.
- Wear glasses or sunglasses to protect your eyes from triggers and put a small amount of Vaseline in each nostril as a barrier to airborne pollutants.
- Wash your hands and rinse your eyes when you come indoors. Wash your hair if you have been exposed to pollen.
- Wear a mask when gardening or mowing your lawn.
- Keep windows in your home closed, as well as those in your car when driving.
- Air condition your home and your car.
- Take frequent "alternate nostril breathing" breaks during the day (see pages 210–11).
- Stay cool but not too cold. Really cold indoor temperatures can aggravate allergy symptoms.

We can't change the weather to suit us, but by studying its effect on our personal health, and in particular our asthmatic condition, we can adapt our lives to its irregularities.

Temperature

We know sudden temperature changes in our surroundings aggravate asthma, but a less recognized contributor to asthma is dramatic temperature variance in the food we eat and drink. Eating food taken directly from the refrigerator or freezer, or drinking icy cold liquids, causes a sudden change of body temperature, which can activate an unexpected response in the bronchial area and possibly trigger an asthma attack. Much the same reaction occurs with liquid or food that is extremely hot. The temperature change may be the trigger for asthma.

You might like to consider the relationship of temperature extremes to your own asthma. If you find this is a triggering factor for you, common sense will tell you to avoid piping hot or freezing cold food and drink.

PART THREE

MANAGEMENT
PLANS AND RECORDS

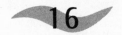

A PLAN FOR MANAGING
ASTHMA

Asthma research organizations and support groups now suggest that everybody with asthma should have a management plan. This is usually quite simple, but sets out clearly what an asthmatic should do to control the condition most successfully. The asthma management plan should also be known to the people the asthmatic lives with – family or friends – so that the plan can be followed by them too, if necessary.

Here is an example of an asthma management plan. Talk to your doctor about the information he or she thinks is important to note in your particular case.

First stage
Realize the extent of your asthma and how it affects you. Make every effort to understand what asthma is. Know your symptoms, what medication you have been prescribed, your asthma history, and lung capacity as measured by a peak flow meter. Keep a diary on the state of your asthma and regularly relay this information to a medical practitioner to ensure that you both monitor your asthma.

Second stage

Ensure you achieve the best lung function you can. Do not underestimate the importance of Controlled Pattern Breathing, exercise and diet.

Third stage

Try to identify what triggers your asthma attacks and where possible avoid them.

Fourth stage

Develop the best program you can to reduce asthma. Use medication that lessens the likelihood of an attack. Consult regularly with your medical practitioner to ensure that you are aware of new medication when it becomes available. Look closely at possible alternative support remedies.

Fifth stage

Ensure that you and your family know the procedures to follow in the event of an attack. For children, ensure the school also knows. Carry with you at all times your medication, instructions about what to do in the event of a severe attack and specific instructions if hospitalization is necessary.

Sixth stage

Evaluate your condition on a regular basis and consult frequently with your health practitioner. Keep up to date with latest asthma developments.

It is always sensible for people with asthma to carry medical details with them, so in the event of a bad attack the correct action can be taken. Overleaf is a sample you may like to use.

ASTHMA INFORMATION CARD
Name:
Address:

Telephone no.:
Regular medication:
Medication during attacks:
Expected peak flow reading:
Peak flow reading requiring extra medication:
If peak flow reading less than   go to
doctor or hospital
Contact person in an emergency:
Telephone no.:
Doctor's name:
Address:

Telephone no.:
Nearest hospital:
Address:

Telephone no.:
Ambulance telephone no.:
Pharmacy:
Address:

Telephone no.:

Monitoring Health Improvement

In order to assess your health and asthma level you need a starting point of your current health. Then by keeping a diary of your daily activities, diet, exercise program, peak-flow readings, supplements taken, asthma attacks and respiratory difficulties, you can compile a monthly report of your progress.

Here is an idea of how you might organize such a record.

Present Health

Date:
Weight:
No. of asthma attacks in previous month:
Medication used over the last month:
Average peak flow reading over last month:
General health   Good/Poor
Known asthma triggers:
Vitamins, herbs, minerals, supplements etc.:
Exercise program   None/Light/Intensive
Any other relevant material:
....

Progressive Record

Date:
Weight:
No. of asthma attacks in previous month:
Medication used over the last month:
Average peak flow reading over last month:
Symptoms:

Sleep disturbance	None/Few/Frequent
Cough	None/Occasional/Frequent
Wheeze	None/Occasional/Frequent
Breathlessness on exertion	None/Mild/Moderate/Severe
General health	Same/Improved/Worse

New asthma triggers:
Diet changes:
Supplements added:
Exercise program   None/Light/Intensive/New
Therapies adopted:
Any other relevant material:
....

For further information about the ideas, suggestions and techniques in this book contact:

Ronald Roberts
P.O. Box 535
Mulgrave North
Victoria 3170
Australia

INDEX
